# Anti-Inflammatory Diet
# Meal Prep

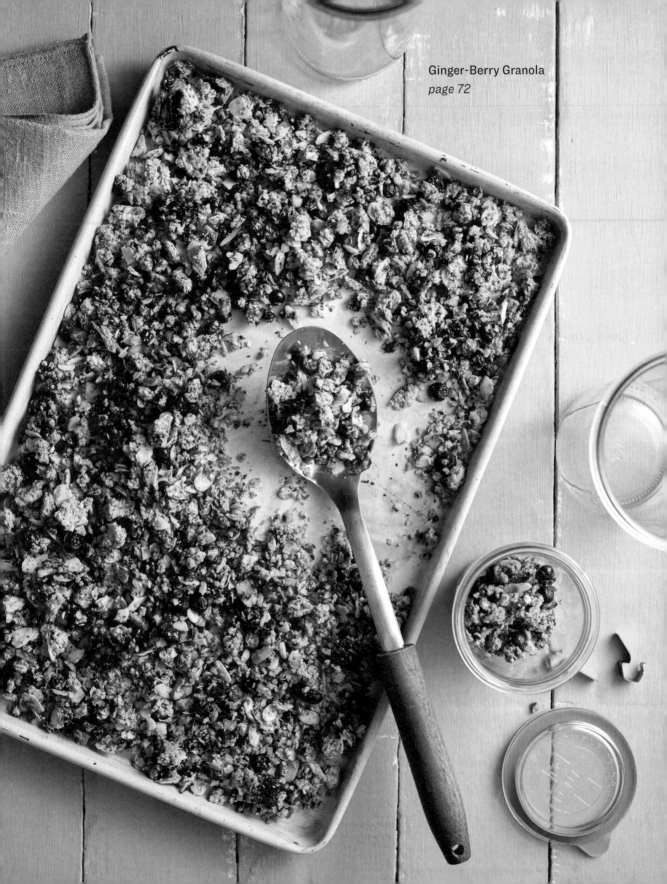

Ginger-Berry Granola
*page 72*

# Anti-Inflammatory Diet Meal Prep

### 6 WEEKLY PLANS AND 80+ RECIPES
### TO SIMPLIFY YOUR HEALING

Ginger Hultin, MS, RDN, CSO

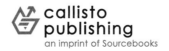
callisto publishing
an imprint of Sourcebooks

Published by Callisto Publishing LLC C/O Sourcebooks LLC
P.O. Box 4410, Naperville, Illinois 60567-4410
(630) 961-3900
callistopublishing.com

Printed and bound in China
OGP 2

To Trevor,
for his unwavering love
and support.

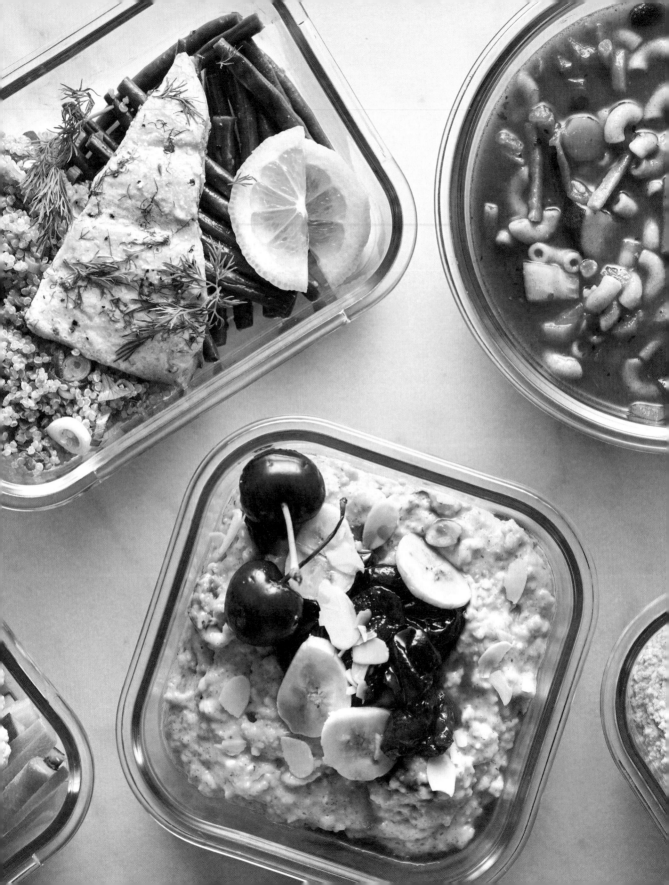

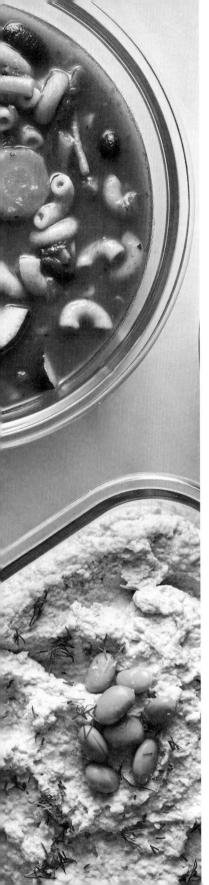

# CONTENTS

||||||||||||||||||||||||||||||||||||||||||||||||||||

# FOREWORD

|||||||||||||||||||||||||||||||||||||||||||||||||||||||||

From the first time I met her in my Nutrition Assessment and Therapy class at Bastyr University, Ginger impressed me as someone who was going to make a difference. She always took on leadership roles and pushed herself, and it has been exciting to watch her grow and succeed over the years. Shortly after completing her master's degree in nutrition, Ginger took on the role of president of the Chicago Affiliate of the Academy of Nutrition and Dietetics and since then has been a regular and trusted contributor to the profession on evidence-based integrative approaches to nutrition.

Ginger regularly contributes to the Academy of Nutrition and Dietetics' *Food & Nutrition Magazine* and is now a national spokesperson for the Academy, contributing countless interviews for print and TV. More recently, she has taught in the clinic and classroom at Bastyr University and the Bastyr Center for Natural Health; spoken at national and international conferences including Today's Dietitian Symposium in Austin, Texas, the Food and Nutrition Conference and Expo in Chicago, and through Catalyst Training Lab in Lebanon, Jordan, and Kuwait; contributed a chapter to a best-selling nutrition textbook, *Krause and Mahan's Food & the Nutrition Care Process* (15th Edition); and has won multiple awards for her work, including the Emerging Dietetic Leader Award from the Washington State Academy of Nutrition and Dietetics in 2020.

Ginger is well connected and keeps her knowledge current on the science of nutrition. She is a prolific writer and blogger, a sought-after consultant, and holds a high standard for her work. In an era where the Internet, bookshelves, and media are full of misinformed "citizen scientists," Ginger provides a trusted, factual, and relatable perspective.

In this book, Ginger will be your guide for building habits and skills to help heal your body and sustain your health. What we eat has a major impact on our health and how quickly we recover from illness—especially inflammatory illness. We are becoming more and more disconnected from the food supply and outsourcing our nourishment and health. Who are we outsourcing to? With the exception of a handful of natural foods companies, the food industry prioritizes convenience, shelf stability, and profit over health. Years ago, a mentor of mine made the statement "If it keeps, you should throw it away"—wise words to live by with our preponderance of highly processed foods.

Meal planning and preparation are essential skills that allow you to reconnect to your food and your health. Ginger developed a passion for this after spending years working with patients who were faced with the daunting challenge of healing from chronic illnesses and learning to nourish themselves through the process. This is an overwhelming task when personal reserves are low. Eating healthy and being nourished doesn't have to be difficult. With the right ingredients and a little planning and knowledge, it can be both empowering and delicious.

This book is full of creative yet simple ideas to help you get organized and motivated to eat better and live a healthier life. Ginger's meal recommendations focus on healthy fats, plant-based proteins, whole grains, herbs and spices, and eating lots more veggies and fruits. Most are naturally gluten- and dairy-free with minimal natural sweeteners—enticing, practical, and anti-inflammatory.

Cheers to Ginger and her latest success!

Kelly Morrow, MS, RDN, FAND
*Associate Professor, Nutrition Clinic Coordinator*
*Department of Nutrition and Exercise Science*
*Bastyr University and the Bastyr Center for Natural Health*

# INTRODUCTION

Inflammation is at the core of illness, and it is a double-edged sword. It can be transient and acute, aiding in healing as a natural part of the injury response. But it can also be unseen and chronic, slowly creating damage across systems in the body. As a longtime registered dietitian nutritionist, I've seen firsthand the damage that chronic, uncontrolled inflammation can do.

My approach to health has always been integrative and holistic. I earned my master's degree in nutrition from Bastyr University in Seattle, Washington, a program known for its natural medicine approach and scientific rigor. I'm a board-certified specialist in oncology nutrition (CSO) and have a background in nutrigenomics, educating clients on how genes interact with both environment and lifestyle to improve or damage health. I've practiced in many clinical settings and have always treated my clients as unique individuals, helping them tackle complex health challenges. I support clients now in my virtual private practice, Champagne Nutrition, located in Seattle, Washington. So many of my clients struggle with inflammation at the root of their health concerns and are looking to make wellness a priority in their busy lives. Health to me has always been about food, movement, sleep, and stress response, and how the systems of the body are working (or not working) together.

Inflammation is linked to chronic illness. Through my work in integrative cancer care, I've seen inflammation fuel weight loss and cachexia to the point that patients were withering away. Levels of inflammation in the body can be measured through the inflammatory marker C-reactive protein, or CRP. Normal levels of CRP are below 3.0 milligrams per liter of blood. In my work, I regularly saw levels above 10, and sometimes upward of 50, indicating severe inflammation.

Cancer can lead to inflammation. In my work with people going through cancer treatment, I saw that sticking to an anti-inflammatory diet, in combination with physical movement, traditional medical treatments, and other integrative support (including stress management and mental health support), helped their CRP levels and other inflammatory markers improve. Some of these people had more energy, and many got well again.

In our busy lives, healthy eating is often put on the back burner. Shopping and cooking can be a burden or a source of additional stress. It's so important to eat healthy when we're sick and our bodies are trying to heal, yet these times are often when we eat worse. The focus of this book is to provide simple, usable resources for you to eat a nourishing, whole foods-based, anti-inflammatory diet without spending excessive time, money, and energy. Meal prepping healthy, anti-inflammatory meals is within your reach, and it can make the difference between sickness and health.

Nutrition is an integral part of healing, whether you have inflammation from cancer, an autoimmune disease, heart disease, diabetes or blood sugar issues, digestive troubles, or any number of other conditions. Nutrition should be a pillar of your healing, and I'm here to support you in your efforts.

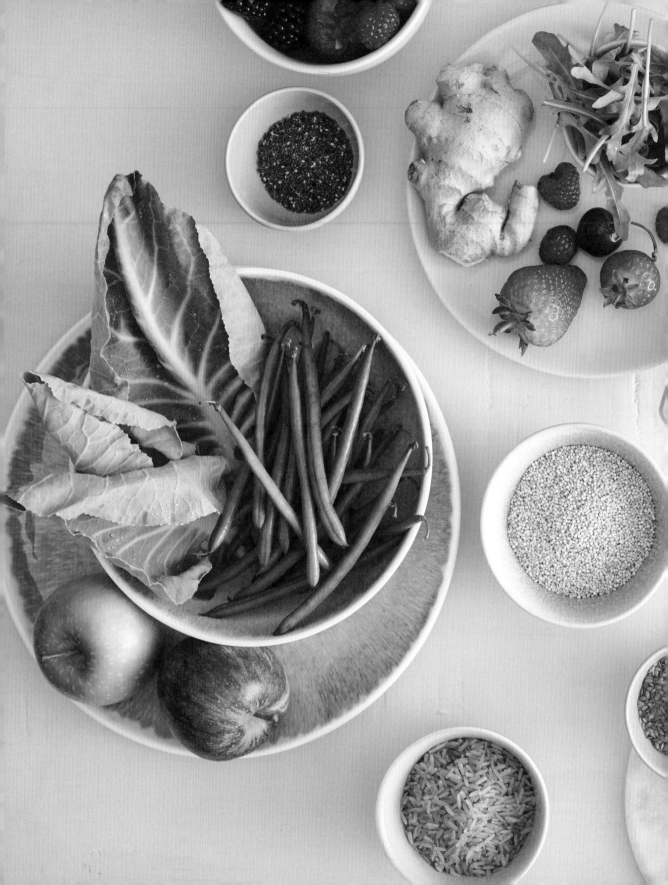

# PART ONE

# The Food and Inflammation Connection

||||||||||||||||||||

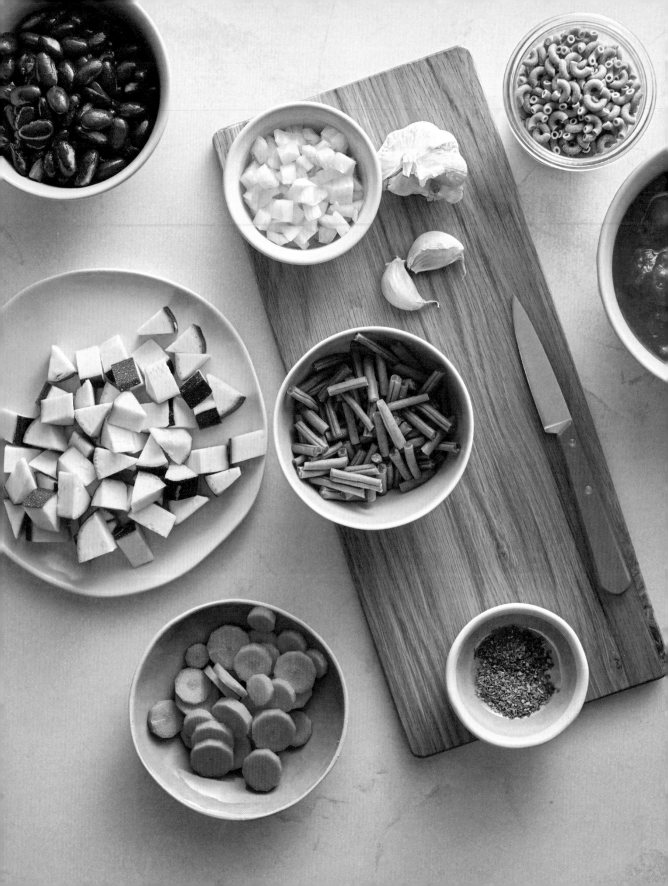

CHAPTER

1

# The Anti-Inflammatory Diet

There's a lot of confusing and conflicting advice about which foods are and are not inflammatory. In this comprehensive guide, I use the most recent and up-to-date research available so you can move forward in your anti-inflammatory diet meal prep with confidence. Eating an anti-inflammatory diet can be simple and easy and can help sustain healthy, balanced eating habits in adults, teens, and children alike.

# Understanding Inflammation

In order to understand the anti-inflammatory diet, it's critical to know what inflammation is and how it works. When it comes to the body, inflammation is a double-edged sword—it can cause pain and discomfort, but it's an important part of healing. When you get a cut, injury, or infection, you'll feel redness, warmth, pain, and swelling around the distressed area. This is an example of acute inflammation, and the symptoms you notice are signs of our body's tissue repair process. The body has specific cells, enzymes, and proteins that lead this chain reaction of events, and as these cells, enzymes, and proteins do their work, they can cause symptoms like fever, fatigue, and loss of appetite. The seasonal flu is a good example of the body's response to internal inflammation. Ideally, the inflammatory process works quickly and effectively, healing the body and returning it to a state of equilibrium.

Unfortunately, there is a second type of inflammation that tends to work against the body rather than for it. This is called chronic inflammation. It occurs when markers of inflammation become chronically elevated, leaving the body in a constant state of irritation. Symptoms of long-term inflammation include chronic fatigue, pain, weight gain (or the inability to lose weight), emotional distress (including anxiety and depression), digestive issues, abdominal pain, and elevated blood pressure or blood sugar levels.

Many diseases can cause chronic inflammation, but so can the way we eat and live our lives. Chronic internal inflammation can be a driving factor for heart disease, cancer, type 2 diabetes, autoimmune diseases, gastrointestinal problems including irritable bowel syndrome and inflammatory bowel diseases, fibromyalgia, and chronic infections. It can be hard to know if you are suffering from a disease that's fueling inflammation in the body or if inflammation is the root cause that needs to be treated. Either way, an anti-inflammatory diet can help reduce the impact of these diseases.

The food you eat every day can either fuel or calm inflammation. This is a major focus of *Anti-Inflammatory Diet Meal Prep*. Because inflammation is such a complex issue, treating it requires taking a comprehensive look at your entire lifestyle to address other factors that can cause stress or irritation to the body, such as exposure to toxins in the environment, lack of sleep, emotional stress, or lack of exercise.

# How Anti-Inflammatory Foods Help the Body Heal

There is a direct link between food and inflammation. A study published in the *Journal of Internal Medicine* found that foods that naturally contain antioxidants can reduce inflammation in the body as well as damage from free radicals. Free radicals are highly reactive molecules with one or more unpaired electrons. When the body has an overload of free radicals, it can enter a state of oxidative stress, and they can begin to damage DNA and healthy cells in the body. Some research, including research published in *Current Opinion in Food Science*, has indicated that the oxidative stress caused by free radicals can be stabilized by antioxidants found in the food you eat. For example, the antioxidant vitamin C, found in broccoli, bell peppers, berries, and citrus, gives its electrons to free radicals in the body, helping prevent damage and leading to reduced inflammation.

There's something special about the anti-inflammatory properties in whole foods. Every fruit, vegetable, grain, and legume has a food matrix: the unique, complex structure of the whole food. An apple, for example, contains water, fiber, and a large variety of vitamins, minerals, and antioxidants. If you juice, dry, or even grind the apple up into pills, you're altering the food matrix and changing the way the apple interacts with the body. This book focuses on preparing food so it remains as close as possible to its whole, unprocessed form.

## NOURISHING FOODS TO ADD

Many foods contain potent anti-inflammatory properties. Foods to support an anti-inflammatory diet include whole grains, legumes, citrus and other fruits and berries, nuts and chia seeds, cocoa, teas, and herbs and spices like ginger, turmeric, and garlic.

**Whole grains.** High-fiber whole grains, including oats, brown rice, and quinoa, are packed with vitamins, minerals, and antioxidants. According to research published in *Nutrition Reviews*, consuming whole grains (as opposed to processed "white" flour products like white bread, pastries, and cookies) could lower inflammatory markers in the body, including CRP. Some people are allergic to or intolerant of wheat or gluten (a protein in wheat, spelt, farro, bulgur, as well as semolina, which is used to make pasta). Because of this, the meal prep in this book will emphasize gluten-free grains. Include a serving of whole grains at least twice per day in your diet.

**Legumes.** Beans, lentils, and soy foods have been found to reduce inflammation in many studies, including ones published in *Nutrition*. They are rich in fiber as well as vitamins, minerals, and many antioxidants. Legumes contain a balance of protein and complex carbohydrates, so they're filling and they'll fuel your energy. Eating whole and fermented soy foods, such as tofu, tempeh, miso, and edamame, can reduce inflammation in the body due to their high fiber and antioxidant content. Current guidelines from the Dietary Guidelines for Americans (DGA) and the American Institute for Cancer Research suggest that soy foods can benefit the cardiovascular system and bone health and may even help prevent some cancers. Include a serving of legumes at least once per day in your diet.

**Fruits and vegetables.** Fruits and vegetables are rich in a variety of antioxidants, including vitamins C and E. The DGAs recommend making them the central part of your diet. According to recent data from the Centers for Disease Control and Prevention, only 12.2 percent and 9.3 percent of Americans are currently meeting their fruit and vegetable intake recommendations, respectively. The different colors of fruits, berries, and vegetables indicate different types of antioxidants. You may have heard the advice to "eat the rainbow," which refers to eating a wide variety of foods to fill the body with different healthy compounds. Include 2 cups of fruit per day and 3 cups of vegetables per day in your diet.

## Staying Hydrated

The body relies on getting enough water to work properly. Water plays a role in every cell in the body; it helps regulate energy levels, and is critical for brain function, skin integrity, and mood. Water makes up the majority of your blood volume, where it helps transport nutrients from the food you eat to the tissues that need it. Water helps detoxify the body, removing waste through sweat, urine, and bowel movements. The National Academy of Medicine (formerly called the Institute of Medicine) has set guidelines for water intake at 2.7 liters per day for adult females and 3.7 liters per day for adult males. Not meeting your fluid needs can cause headaches, increase the risk of kidney stones (due to low urine volume), and even impair attention and cognition.

When planning your weekly meals, make sure that you set water intake goals. Fill a pitcher of water and keep it in your refrigerator or on your counter to keep it at the front of your mind. Purchase a reusable water bottle and set goals for how many times you need to refill it per day. You can also try infusing your water with fruit, vegetables, or herbs for more flavor and anti-inflammatory support.

**Nuts, seeds, and omega-3s.** Nuts and seeds contain many important anti-inflammatory nutrients including antioxidant vitamin E and heart-healthy unsaturated fatty acids. Some nuts and seeds, such as chia, flax, and walnuts, contain a unique type of healthy fat called omega-3 fatty acids, which according to research in *The American Journal of Clinical Nutrition* and other journals has been shown to lower inflammation in the body. Cold-water fish like salmon and halibut are another source of omega-3s. Include a portion of nuts and seeds daily and omega-3-rich fish twice per week in your diet.

**Cocoa.** Chocolate, specifically antioxidant-rich cocoa, has been shown to have anti-inflammatory properties, according to research published in *Nutrients* and other journals. It's important to incorporate pure dark chocolate rather than prepared chocolate with added sugars and saturated fat. Include cocoa in your diet three to four times per week.

**Herbs, spices, and tea.** Herbs and spices are an important part of an anti-inflammatory diet. Foods like garlic, cinnamon, and turmeric should be staples in your pantry. Ginger is an herb that has been specifically associated with calming inflammation. Not only does it soothe the stomach and reduce nausea, but studies, including one published in the *Journal of Medicinal Food*, have shown that it can significantly reduce levels of CRP. Tea is another antioxidant-rich ingredient that has been shown to calm inflammation in the body, according to research published in *Brain, Behavior, and Immunity*. You'll see green tea used in this book's recipes as well. Incorporate herbs, spices, and tea multiple times per day in your diet.

## INFLAMMATORY FOODS TO AVOID

There are several types of food that should generally be avoided or else greatly reduced, because they cause inflammation in the body. Some research, including a study published in *The American Journal of Clinical Nutrition*, has indicated a link between inflammation and processed foods, alcohol, trans fats, an imbalanced ratio of omega-6s to omega-3s, and sugar. Some people also have allergies or intolerances that cause an inflammatory response to certain foods, such as gluten, dairy, and nightshade vegetables.

**Highly processed foods.** "Processed" food refers to any food that has been altered from its natural state. For instance, even precut vegetables are "processed." In this book, though, when I refer to processed foods to avoid, I'm referring to highly processed or ultraprocessed foods—ones that have been *significantly* altered from their original form. Foods that contain refined "white" grains and flours (stripped of fiber and nutrients), added sugars, artificial colors, flavors, stabilizers, and other chemicals have become an increasingly normal part of the standard American diet. Ultraprocessing makes food shelf-stable for sale in stores and restaurants, but it can also make food higher in calories and lower in fiber and other nutrients that the body needs for health. Fried foods are often highly processed, so I'll make suggestions throughout this book for how to substitute healthier alternatives for fried foods.

**Alcohol.** Alcohol intake beyond current guidelines listed in the DGAs—one drink per day for women and two drinks per day for men—can lead to inflammation in the body, specifically in the gastrointestinal tract and liver. If you need to maintain an anti-inflammatory diet for your health, it is worth considering ceasing drinking or drinking only on rare occasions.

**Trans fats and fat imbalance.** Pro-inflammatory trans fats have been banned in the US, after the FDA found a strong link between trans fats, inflammation, and heart disease. Awareness about the risk of trans fats has improved, but you can still find them in small amounts, disguised on food labels as "partially hydrogenated oils." Trans fats should be strictly avoided. An imbalance of omega-6 to omega-3 fatty acids may also fuel inflammation, according to research published in the *American Journal of Kidney Diseases*. The standard American diet tends to have a surplus of omega-6s, so an anti-inflammatory diet will require adding in omega-3s to create balance.

**Sugar and sugar substitutes.** Current guidelines on added sugar are clear: Per the American Heart Association (AHA), added sugar should be no more than 10 percent of your daily calories (25 grams for women, 36 grams for men). However, an AHA study found that Americans consume on average nearly 80 grams per day. AHA research suggests that limiting sugar intake to the recommended amount could lead to a drop in inflammation levels. A diet rich in whole foods is virtually devoid of added sugars (and sugar substitutes, which are usually found only in ultraprocessed foods).

**Wheat and gluten.** Minimally processed whole grains are generally anti-inflammatory, but some people experience inflammation after eating wheat or gluten if they have an allergy or intolerance. Whole wheat is high in fiber, vitamins, and minerals, but many people with autoimmune disorders, including celiac disease, cannot tolerate it. It may be an interesting experiment to see if you feel better after removing wheat or gluten from your diet.

**Dairy.** Though studies on the link between dairy and inflammation have mixed findings, there is some evidence of a link between proteins in dairy and autoimmune diseases, such as type 1 diabetes (research has been published in *Diabetologia*). Other research has indicated the anti-inflammatory properties specifically of fermented dairy (yogurt, kefir, and sour cream) and low-fat dairy. Dairy products are used only rarely in this book, and nondairy substitutes are always provided. Dairy products are a major source of protein and minerals, so I've taken care to supplement those nutrients in other ways. I often recommend soy milk, which is higher in protein and antioxidants than other nondairy milks.

**Nightshades.** Some people with autoimmune diseases or other inflammatory conditions avoid nightshade vegetables, including tomatoes, eggplants, white potatoes, paprika, cayenne pepper, and bell peppers, for fear that their solanine content, a compound found in these plants, could increase inflammation. Claims that solanine in nightshades causes inflammation have not been verified; in fact, much evidence has pointed to the fact that these foods are anti-inflammatory. However, since some people may be sensitive or allergic to nightshade vegetables, this book uses them in recipes minimally.

For your convenience, here is an at-a-glance table on what foods to enjoy, minimize, and avoid. You can and should interpret this to fit what you already know about your own body.

| Foods to Enjoy | Foods to Minimize | Foods to Avoid |
|---|---|---|
| Whole grains (quinoa, oats, brown rice) | Alcohol (beer, wine, spirits) | Highly processed foods |
| Legumes (beans, lentils, whole and fermented soy foods) | Wheat and gluten | Trans fats |
| Fruits and vegetables (leafy greens, cruciferous vegetables, squash, onions, carrots, peas, green beans, apples, oranges, stone fruit, berries, tropical fruit, and melons) | Dairy | Added sugars |
| Nuts and seeds (tree nuts, sesame, chia, flax, and sunflower seeds) and omega-3-rich foods (wild salmon and other cold-water fish, such as halibut, trout, and herring) | | Sugar substitutes, artificial colors and flavors, and fried foods—these are usually indicators of ultraprocessed foods |
| Cocoa | | |
| Herbs and spices (ginger, garlic, turmeric, basil, oregano, cumin, thyme, cinnamon) and teas (green and herbal) | | |

# Following an Anti-Inflammatory Diet

As you transition to an anti-inflammatory diet, your foundation should be increasing foods you already enjoy while trying new foods and maintaining flexibility in your diet. Simple swaps to add in healthy fats and prioritizing fruits and vegetables can have a big effect on inflammation in the body.

**Increase foods you enjoy.** Adapting to an anti-inflammatory diet shouldn't require turning your world upside down. Focus on increasing the anti-inflammatory foods you already enjoy, and the other foods will fall away naturally.

**Keep an open mind.** Try new foods and prepare foods you didn't previously enjoy in new ways. There's no need to eat plain, unseasoned vegetables, beans, or grains—the herbs and spices used in these recipes will help maximize flavor.

**Meet your own needs and preferences.** The recipes and meal-prep plans in this book are meant to be flexible. If you have specific food allergies or preferences, make adjustments to suit your needs. I'll offer substitutions and tips along the way so that you can adapt easily.

**Swap in healthy fats.** Cook with fats and oils that come from natural sources. Use fats like olive oil and coconut oil and add in plenty of omega-3-rich ingredients, such as chia and flax seeds, walnuts, and fatty fish.

**Rethink snacks.** Simplify your snack options by choosing fruits, vegetables, nuts and seeds, and homemade dips and spreads. This book includes plenty of snack-prep plans, so there's no need to purchase packaged chips or crackers.

**Include fruits and veggies in every meal.** In an anti-inflammatory diet plan, your meals will revolve around produce. Stocking up on fresh and frozen fruits and veggies will help you include them in every meal and snack so you can meet your daily goals with ease.

## Lifestyle Choices That Support Your Healing

Calming inflammation in the body requires more than changing your diet. The best health results will come from a holistic approach. By focusing on an anti-inflammatory lifestyle, you can create an environment that will support you working to lower chronic inflammation permanently. Here are some things you can do to support your positive dietary changes.

**Exercise daily.** There is evidence of a direct link between increased exercise and decreased inflammation in the body. The US Department of Health and Human Services' recommended guidelines for physical activity are 150 minutes of moderate aerobic activity or 75 minutes of vigorous activity, plus two days of strength training every week.

**Reduce stress.** Stress management is a critical piece of body wellness. Physical stress (like chronic pain) and mental or emotional stress (from family or work dynamics, social difficulties, or chronic depression and anxiety) may increase inflammation. There are many ways to reduce stress, including connecting with friends and family, spending quality time alone, getting outside, exercising, meditating, deep breathing, or getting mental health support.

**Focus on sleep.** Lack of sleep may lead to inflammation as well as increased body weight and lowered immune response. Making sleep a priority is one of the most critical things you can do for your health.

**Heal the gut.** Research continues to improve our understanding of the importance of a healthy microbiome (bacteria) in the digestive tract, especially the lower intestines and colon. Preliminary research indicates that a high-fiber, anti-inflammatory diet may help foster a healthy digestive tract.

**Reduce toxic exposure.** Buildup of toxic substances like mercury, lead, air pollutants, BPA, dioxins, phthalates, and others may create an inflammatory toxic load in some people. Exposure to cigarettes, cigars, or e-cigs can also lead to inflammation. While it's nearly impossible in the modern world to eliminate toxins completely, it's important to take steps to reduce exposure.

# Benefits of Eating an Anti-Inflammatory Diet

Whether or not you have chronic inflammation, eating an anti-inflammatory diet can benefit your health. This is because an anti-inflammatory diet is made up of foods that are, well, healthy! It maximizes nutrient-dense foods full of fiber, vitamins, minerals, and antioxidants. For this reason, an anti-inflammatory diet can benefit people of all ages with all types of health needs.

If you do experience chronic inflammation in the body and are suffering from associated diseases or fatigue, the anti-inflammatory diet can change your life. You may see your test results for CRP or other inflammatory markers improve. You may notice improved energy levels, have less chronic pain, experience fewer symptom flare-ups, and sleep more peacefully. You may find you can resume doing things you loved but had to give up.

As you grow accustomed to eating anti-inflammatory foods, you may feel it become easy and effortless. You might feel more in control of your schedule and feel positive about what you're putting in your body. I recommend trying this meal plan for four to six weeks and tracking your symptoms so you can get a better idea of the changes you experience.

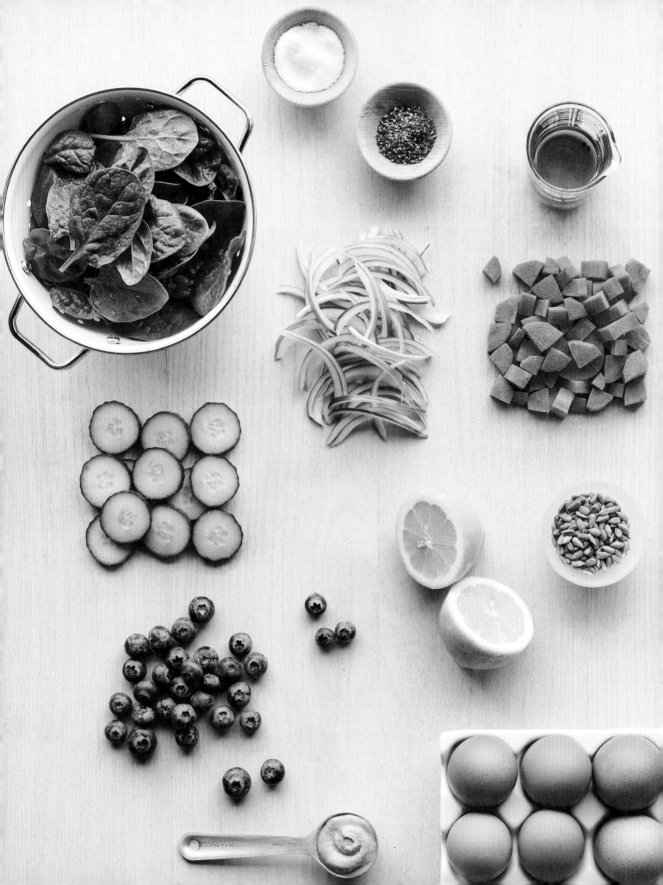

Garlic-Herb Marinated Tofu
*page 95*

CHAPTER

**2**

# Meal-Prep Essentials

Whether you're new to meal prepping or not, prepping large batches of healthy food will make your life easier. When you open the refrigerator or freezer, you'll have lots of healthy options ready to go, eliminating your reliance on fast food and unhealthy convenience snacks. This chapter will prepare you to start meal prepping. I'll go over a plan for how to make meal prep doable, provide information on storage and equipment, and explain how the recipes are structured and why they offer anti-inflammatory benefits.

# Why Meal Prep?

Meal prepping is designed specifically to make eating healthier easier and to cut back on time spent shopping for, cooking, and preparing meals. It can sometimes be confusing to start, but following the prep plans in the next chapters will make things clear, simple, and easy to build upon. Soon, you'll get back time, money, and your health.

**Make healthy easy.** Many of us rush to work or school in the morning and choose fast food or unhealthy convenience options—and sometimes we skip breakfast altogether. With a meal-prep plan, you'll always have a healthy option to grab, even when you're short on time.

**Remove the guesswork from anti-inflammatory eating.** It can be a lot of work to look up recipes and research foods that calm inflammation. This book does the work for you. These recipes align with up-to-date knowledge of anti-inflammatory foods, and they're designed for you to adjust ingredients to fit your personal needs.

**Reduce stress.** Figuring out breakfast, lunch, and dinner every day for yourself and others is a huge amount of work. By following a meal plan that's already made for you, you'll be able to put meals on the table without the mental gymnastics.

**Save money.** Planning ahead, shopping only for what you need, buying whole, unprocessed foods, and reusing ingredients will save you money. The meal-prep plans in this book include shopping lists to help you cut back on expensive packaged foods and impulse buys.

**Save time.** This book will teach you to cook more food in fewer batches. Once you cook recipes for the week, you can be completely done with your prep, saving hours of time every day.

# Six-Step Prep

There are simple steps you can take to set yourself up for meal-prep success. Planning ahead for your prep days, grocery shopping, and preparing and packaging your meals in effective ways will save you time in the long run.

1. **Choose your prep day(s).** It doesn't matter what day you choose to meal prep, but you'll need about 4 hours to cook your recipes and divide them into their containers for the week. The plans in this book are designed to last 5 days. For instance, you

could prep meals on Sunday for Monday through Friday. If you have a different schedule, shift the plan to suit your needs.

2. **Make a plan.** The first 6 weeks of meal-prep plans are laid out for you. After that, you'll be ready to plan your own meal or swap recipes into the existing structure. Set aside 30 minutes to 1 hour to make your plan each week, and consider doing it a day or two before your prep day so you have time to buy groceries. Use the prep charts in this book as a template.

3. **Go grocery shopping.** Once you have a plan, write a shopping list. To speed up shopping, group your ingredients by where you'll find them in the store, such as the bulk aisle, herbs and spices area, dry goods, refrigerated items, fresh produce, frozen foods, and so on.

4. **Prepare and cook.** Before you start cooking, take out the ingredients and kitchen tools you'll need for each recipe. Once everything is set up, make a cooking plan. Check the timing of the recipes and see which makes sense to prepare first. As you start to do this, it will get easier. For example, you can make a sauce while a sheet pan meal is roasting. You can chop similar ingredients all at once; if three recipes use parsley, chop the total amount at once and portion it out per recipe.

5. **Portion and pack.** Once your meals are prepped, review the weekly plan and the serving sizes, and set all your containers out on the counter. Portion the meals into their containers according to the serving size on the meal plan. Label and date as needed, and store them in the refrigerator or freezer so they're easy to see.

6. **Grab and go.** Consider getting a thermal lunch bag and investing in reusable utensils for breakfast or lunch on the go. Meal prepping won't work if you forget to bring your food with you!

# Kitchen Equipment

Having a few simple, affordable kitchen tools on hand can make meal prep much easier. Organize your cupboards so these items are easy to find and access.

**Blender.** From smoothies to sauces, a blender is an essential kitchen tool. Make sure your blender is easy to use and clean, and keep it where you can access it easily.

**Cutting boards.** You'll be chopping a lot of fruit and veggies, so having a series of cutting boards is key. Large, sturdy plastic boards can be easily cleaned and can go in the dishwasher.

**Knives.** Invest in high-quality chef's and paring knives. Quality knives are safer, quicker, and easier to use.

**Measuring cups and spoons.** Following recipes is easier when you have measuring cups and spoons. You can also use them to help measure portion sizes.

**Mixing bowls.** A set of bowls is critical for meal prep, allowing you to multitask in the kitchen. Choose a set that offers a variety of sizes, but have at least two large bowls on hand for the large quantities of food you'll be preparing.

**Pot.** A soup pot is useful for big batches of soups or stews and for cooking pasta.

**Saucepan.** A 7-inch (or 3-quart) saucepan with a lid is a versatile tool for cooking grains and sauces.

**Sheet pan or rimmed baking sheet.** Since you'll be prepping larger portions of food, a good baking sheet (or two) that has sides is a critical tool.

**Skillet.** A high-quality 12- to 14-inch pan with a lid will help you cook large quantities of food.

**Spoons and spatulas.** I recommend a set of wooden spoons as well as a large and small spatula to allow you to prep and transfer food easily.

## STORAGE ESSENTIALS

The key to successful meal prepping is having the right storage. Since you'll be prepping 5 breakfasts, 5 lunches, and 5 dinners per week per person, you'll need at least 15 containers of various types and sizes. I always recommend airtight containers.

**Single and multicompartment.** Some recipes in this book must be stored in different compartments—in the style of a bento box—to keep individual ingredients fresh until you eat. Other recipes can be stored in single-serving containers. Keep both single and multicompartment containers on hand.

**Stackable/nestable.** Pantry, refrigerator, and freezer organization is vital to efficient meal prepping. Consider a set of matching stackable containers that can fit on top of one another, especially if you're low on kitchen space.

**Glass.** The gold standard of meal prep is a good glass container with a secure lid. You can see through them to view the contents, they won't stain, and they're microwave- and dishwasher-safe. Consider investing in glass containers (some are designed for meal prep) as well as glass jars with screw-top lids for soups, oats, or dressings.

**Plastic, if necessary.** Thick plastic containers can be used for meal-prep storage, but not all plastic is food-safe. Plastic containers should be designed specifically for food storage, dishwasher-safe, and marked "BPA-free," meaning they do not contain the compound bisphenol A, which can seep into food.

# Long-Term Meal-Prep Success

Sticking with meal prep long-term involves changing your habits and committing to a new way of prepping, shopping, and cooking. Cooking in batches, reusing ingredients, freezing foods, and proper reheating will make it easier to follow a plan.

**Cook in batches.** Things that you used to cook every night, like a pot of rice or quinoa, you'll now cook in larger batches just once a week. Instead of 1 sweet potato, you'll cook 5 at once. Instead of 2 servings of rice, you'll cook 6. Batch-cooking takes the stress out of cooking every single night.

**Reuse ingredients.** There are anti-inflammatory staple ingredients throughout this book that can be cooked in batches and reused in many recipes. Cooked quinoa shows up in breakfast, lunch, and dinner recipes. A sauce for one recipe can work well in another. Use your favorite meal-prep ingredients and recipes to create a weekly plan that you look forward to.

**Know what (and what not) to freeze.** Not all foods can be frozen. For example, fresh leafy greens (like lettuce and spinach), chickpeas, and pasta salads won't freeze well. Salad dressings and some other sauces will change texture if frozen. In contrast, soups and stews freeze easily and can be stored frozen for up to 3 months.

**Learn how to reheat.** If a food is frozen, it must be thawed first before it can be reheated in the microwave or on the stovetop. Integrate this into your planning by moving frozen foods to the refrigerator to thaw the day before your prep day. Thawed foods generally last in the refrigerator for up to 3 days before serving.

## Shortcuts to Even Easier Prep

Meal prepping for an anti-inflammatory diet takes some getting used to. It requires setting aside dedicated time and committing to a new way of preparing and cooking food. To make it easier on yourself, look for shortcuts. For instance, you don't need to completely forgo every type of convenience food. Canned beans are an affordable, convenient, and healthy option. Frozen fruits and vegetables retain their nutrient content as well as, or better than, the fresh versions. Here are some tips that can make a big impact on the ease of prepping and the time it takes you to prep, without sacrificing flavor or anti-inflammatory properties:

- Buy prewashed, bagged, or packaged salad greens that are already chopped. These options make salads quick to prep.

- Choose frozen fruits such as blueberries, strawberries, raspberries, and cherries. They're often more affordable than their fresh counterparts.

- Buy tomato sauce in a can or jar. Read the nutrition facts to ensure there's minimal or no added sugar.

- Canned beans are affordable and faster to cook than dried beans, and you can rinse them to remove excess salt from brine. Look for BPA-free cans or boxes.

- Purchase jars of minced garlic to save time mincing fresh garlic for these recipes.

# About the Recipes and Meal-Prep Plans

The meal-prep plans in the next chapters are designed to get you started with the meal-prep lifestyle and help you begin to incorporate anti-inflammatory foods into your diet. You'll see plans laid out with breakfast, lunch, and dinner, Monday through Friday. I also include snacks that you can use between meals. If you can, I suggest you meet with a registered dietitian to learn more about what calorie needs you should aim for. Some people will need more or less than what is represented in the book.

Weeks 1 and 2 focus on eliminating highly processed foods and replacing them with anti-inflammatory whole foods that are easy to prep and store. Weeks 3 and 4 will help you increase fruit and vegetable intake. Weeks 5 and 6 include recipes that highlight foods packed with antioxidants and other healthy nutrients to calm inflammation.

The first two weeks keep the planning very simple, with recipes for breakfast, lunch, and dinner. The next two weeks introduce options to rotate meal choices for dinner, and the last two weeks offer further variation. These meal-prep plans are not set in stone; they are only designed to provide a structure to work within. My hope is that, with practice, you'll be able to design meal-prep plans on your own.

Every meal-prep plan includes a shopping list, instructions for prepping and cooking, and recipes. If you want to keep things simple, you can use these plans over and over. Part 3 (page 81) has even more recipes so you can begin making your custom meal prep plans and exploring more ways to prepare anti-inflammatory meals.

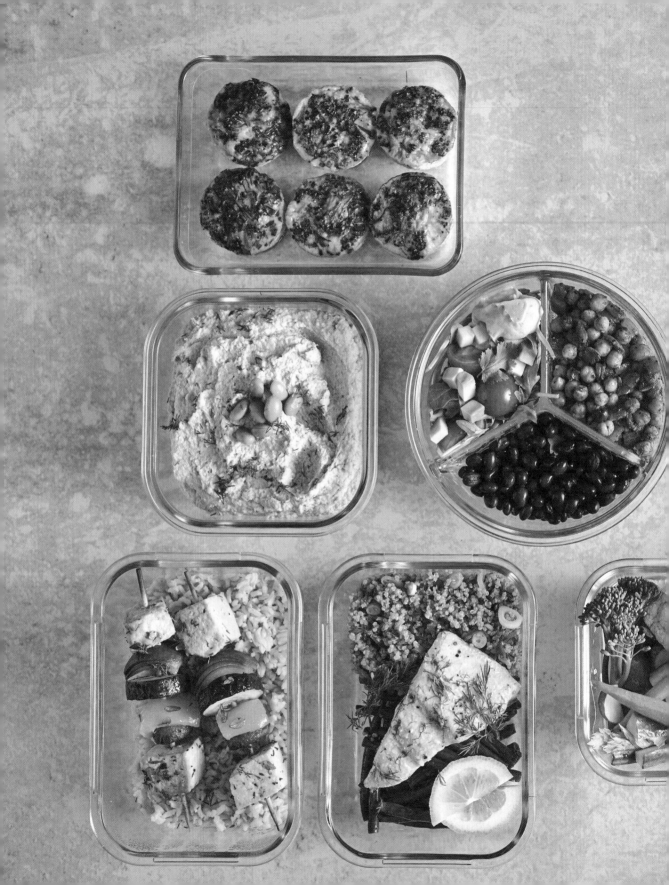

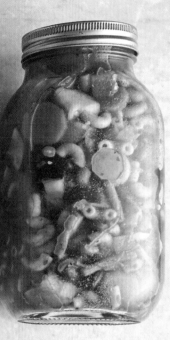

# PART TWO

# Meal-Prep Plans for Anti-Inflammatory Eating

||||||||||||||||||||||

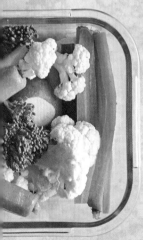

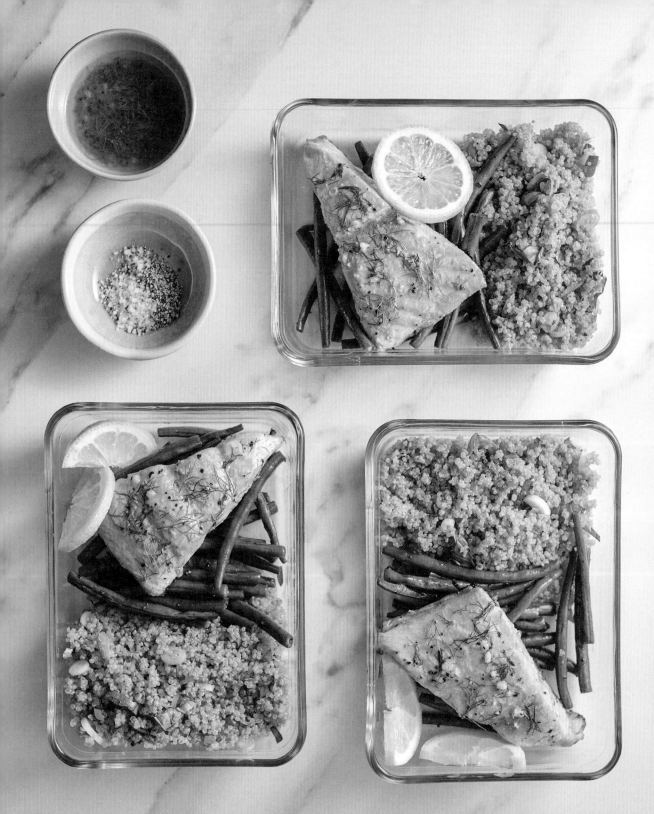

Salmon with Savory Herbed Quinoa
and String Beans
*page 38*

# CHAPTER 3

# Weeks 1 and 2 Meal Prep

Let's keep Weeks 1 and 2 simple! Breaking up with processed foods is easier when you're prepared with breakfast, lunch, dinner, and snacks. When you have a week of healthy, anti-inflammatory meals prepped and ready to go, you won't need to rely on processed foods anymore. In Weeks 1 and 2, I have just one recipe for breakfast, one for lunch, and one for dinner. There are lots of ways to add variety later on, but for now, we'll start with three recipes to plan, shop, and prep for. You'll soon realize how much less time you're spending on meals from the very beginning, and the anti-inflammatory ingredients will support your health, nourish your body, and start to calm your system down.

||||||||||||||||||||||||||||||||||||||||||||||||

# Breaking Up with Processed Foods Week 1

| | BREAKFAST | LUNCH | DINNER |
|---|---|---|---|
| **DAY 1** | Overnight Oats with Cinnamon, Berries, and Soy Milk | Lemony Split Pea Soup | Tempeh Taco Salad |
| **DAY 2** | Overnight Oats with Cinnamon, Berries, and Soy Milk | Tempeh Taco Salad | Lemony Split Pea Soup |
| **DAY 3** | Overnight Oats with Cinnamon, Berries, and Soy Milk | Lemony Split Pea Soup | Tempeh Taco Salad |
| **DAY 4** | Overnight Oats with Cinnamon, Berries, and Soy Milk | Tempeh Taco Salad | Lemony Split Pea Soup |
| **DAY 5** | Overnight Oats with Cinnamon, Berries, and Soy Milk | Lemony Split Pea Soup | Tempeh Taco Salad |

**Snacks as needed:** Cantaloupe or honeydew melon

## SHOPPING LIST

### Produce

- Bananas (3)
- Blueberries or strawberries (2½ cups), fresh or frozen
- Carrots, medium (3)
- Celery (3 stalks)
- Cilantro (1 bunch)
- Garlic (1 head)
- Lemons (2)
- Lettuce, romaine (3 heads)
- Limes (4)
- Melon, cantaloupe or honeydew (1 large or 5 cups chopped), for snacking
- Onions, yellow, medium (2)
- Potatoes, golden, medium (2)
- Scallions (1 bunch)
- Turmeric root (2 inches) or ground turmeric (1 teaspoon)

## Dairy and Dairy Alternatives

- Soy milk, unsweetened, but vanilla is okay (½ gallon)

## Protein

- Beans, pinto, 1 (15.5-ounce) can
- Chia seeds (5 tablespoons)
- Split peas, yellow (2 cups)
- Tempeh, 2 (8-ounce) packages

## Canned/Bottled/Pantry

- Basil, dried
- Broth, vegetable (1 quart/32 fluid ounces)
- Chili powder
- Cinnamon, ground
- Cumin, ground
- Garlic powder
- Honey
- Mustard, Dijon
- Oats, old-fashioned rolled (2½ cups)
- Oil, olive
- Onion powder
- Oregano, dried
- Peppercorns, black (in a grinder) or ground black pepper
- Salt
- Thyme, dried
- Turmeric, ground, if not using fresh
- Vanilla extract
- Vinegar, apple cider

## EQUIPMENT

- Blender, immersion or stand (for the soup)
- Bowls: 1 large, 1 medium, 1 small
- Chef's knife and paring knife
- Cutting boards
- Fine-mesh sieve
- Large pot
- Large skillet
- Measuring cups and spoons
- Spatulas
- Storage containers: 15 medium, 5 small
- Storage jars with screw-top lids (5)
- Whisks
- Wooden spoons

## STEP-BY-STEP PREP

|||||||||||||||||||||||||||||||||||||||||||||||||||||||||||||||||||||||

1. Follow step 1 and the beginning of step 2 of the **Lemony Split Pea Soup** (page 30) until the soup is simmering.

2. While the soup simmers, move on to the **Overnight Oats with Cinnamon, Berries, and Soy Milk** (page 29). Follow all the steps, including the storage instructions.

3. For the remainder of the time that the soup is simmering, follow steps 1 through 3 for the **Tempeh Taco Salad** (page 31). And set the tempeh aside to cool. By this point, the split pea soup should be close to done cooking. Once the split peas are soft, move on to step 3 of the soup recipe to blend it and set it aside to cool.

4. Once the tempeh taco salad ingredients are cool, follow steps 4 through 6 of the taco recipe to make the dressing and separate the cooked tempeh mixture, chopped lettuce, and dressing into separate containers and refrigerate.

5. Divide the cooled split pea soup into 5 medium containers and store in the refrigerator.

# Overnight Oats with Cinnamon, Berries, and Soy Milk

**DAIRY-FREE • GLUTEN-FREE • NIGHTSHADE-FREE • NUT-FREE • VEGAN**
**Makes** 5 servings
**Prep time:** 10 minutes, plus overnight

These overnight oats make use of several anti-inflammatory ingredients. Oats contain fiber compounds that can strengthen the immune system. Cinnamon and berries contain potent antioxidant properties, and soy milk offers protein to keep you energized and lots of antioxidants.

2½ cups old-fashioned rolled oats

5 tablespoons chia seeds

2 teaspoons ground cinnamon

5 cups unsweetened soy milk

5 teaspoons pure vanilla extract

3 bananas, mashed

2½ cups fresh or frozen blueberries or strawberries

1. In a large bowl, combine the oats, chia seeds, and cinnamon. Add the soy milk, vanilla, and mashed banana. Whisk to combine and set aside for 10 minutes until the mixture thickens slightly.
2. Portion 1½ cups of the mixture into each of 5 glass jars with screw-top lids. Top each jar with ½ cup of berries, screw on the lids, and place in the refrigerator.

✳ **Storage:** Store the prepared overnight oats in the refrigerator. Enjoy oats cold or hot (microwaved for 1 to 2 minutes). As the oats absorb more liquid with time, you may need to add a tablespoon or two of soy milk the final 2 days of the week.

✳ **Ingredient tip:** Oats are naturally gluten-free but are often processed in facilities that also process gluten-containing foods like wheat flour. If you have celiac disease or need to strictly avoid gluten, make sure to purchase oats labeled "gluten-free."

✳ **Substitution tip:** If you're soy-free, feel free to replace the soy milk with oat or almond milk.

*Per serving: Calories: 433; Total Fat: 9g; Saturated Fat: 1g; Protein: 15g; Total Carbohydrates: 75g; Fiber: 15g; Sugar: 15g; Cholesterol: 0mg*

# Lemony Split Pea Soup

**DAIRY-FREE · GLUTEN-FREE · NUT-FREE · SOY-FREE · VEGAN**
**Makes** 5 servings
**Prep time:** 20 minutes · **Cook time:** 1 hour 30 minutes

This fresh take on split pea soup is meat-free but super filling due to the high amount of fiber and protein in the ingredients. The lemon provides anti-inflammatory antioxidants like vitamin C and, along with other herbs and spices in this soup, brightens up the flavors. If you feel so inclined, make a double batch—this soup freezes well!

2 tablespoons olive oil
1 medium yellow
   onion, diced
3 celery stalks, diced
3 medium carrots, diced
2 garlic cloves, minced
1 teaspoon ground
   turmeric, or
   1 tablespoon grated
   fresh turmeric root
1 teaspoon dried thyme
½ teaspoon freshly
   ground black pepper
2 cups yellow split
   peas, rinsed
2 medium golden
   potatoes, diced
1¼ teaspoons salt
4 cups vegetable broth
2 cups water, divided
Juice of 2 lemons

1. In a large pot, heat the oil over medium heat. Once warm, add the onion, celery, and carrots and cook, stirring frequently, for about 10 minutes, until the vegetables are soft and the onions are translucent.
2. Add the garlic, turmeric, thyme, pepper, split peas, potatoes, salt, broth, and 1 cup of water. Increase the heat to medium-high and bring to a boil, then reduce the heat to medium, cover, and simmer for 45 to 50 minutes, until the split peas are soft.
3. Stir in the remaining 1 cup of water. Remove 2 cups of soup and blend in a stand blender, then mix it back into the unblended soup. (Alternatively, use an immersion blender.) Stir in the lemon juice. Set the soup aside to cool.
4. Divide the soup among 5 medium storage containers.

\* **Storage:** Store in the refrigerator for up to 5 days. Freeze the soup for up to 6 months. To serve, microwave the soup for 2 to 3 minutes, stirring every 30 seconds, until hot.

\* **Substitution tip:** Use low-sodium broth if you prefer. This anti-inflammatory diet is naturally low in sodium, so I generally use regular-sodium broth for its flavor.

*Per serving:* *Calories: 434; Total Fat: 7g; Saturated Fat: 1g; Protein: 21g; Total Carbohydrates: 76g; Fiber: 24g; Sugar: 12g; Cholesterol: 0mg*

# Tempeh Taco Salad

**DAIRY-FREE · GLUTEN-FREE · NUT-FREE · VEGETARIAN**
**Makes** 5 servings
**Prep time:** 30 minutes · **Cook time:** 10 minutes

Tempeh, a fermented soy product, makes incredible taco "meat." Seasoned the same way you would ground beef or turkey, tempeh provides anti-inflammatory benefits. It's fermented, so it may support digestion, and contains fiber and antioxidants not found in meat.

⅓ cup Anti-Inflammatory Multiuse Spice Blend (page 84)

2 (8-ounce) packages tempeh

5 to 7 tablespoons water

2 tablespoons olive oil

½ yellow onion, diced

1 (15.5-ounce) can pinto beans, drained and rinsed

Honey-Lime Vinaigrette with Fresh Herbs (page 85)

3 heads romaine lettuce, roughly chopped

1. Make the spice blend as directed.
2. In a medium bowl, use a wooden spoon or your fingertips to crumble the tempeh into very small pieces. Add the spice blend and 3 to 4 tablespoons of water. Stir to combine, coating the tempeh thoroughly.
3. In a large skillet, heat the olive oil over medium heat. Add the onion and cook for 4 to 5 minutes, or until soft. Add the tempeh crumble mixture and 2 to 3 tablespoons of additional water, if needed, to prevent sticking. Stir well before adding the pinto beans, and cook, stirring occasionally for 4 to 6 minutes, until all the ingredients are hot. Set it aside to cool.
4. Prepare the vinaigrette as directed. Portion the dressing evenly into 5 separate small containers (about ¼ cup each).
5. Divide the chopped romaine evenly into 5 separate medium containers (about 1½ cups each).
6. Divide the cooled tempeh mixture evenly into 5 separate medium containers.

∗ **Storage:** Store the containers of tempeh mixture alongside the lettuce and dressing in the refrigerator for up to 5 days. To assemble, pour the dressing over the lettuce, then top with tempeh (microwaved separately for 2 minutes, if desired).

∗ **Substitution tip:** If you're avoiding nightshades, eliminate the chili powder in the spice blend recipe.

*Per serving: Calories: 388; Total Fat: 17g; Saturated Fat: 3g; Protein: 27g; Total Carbohydrates: 40g; Fiber: 14g; Sugar: 6g; Cholesterol: 0mg*

# Breaking Up with Processed Foods Week 2

|  | BREAKFAST | LUNCH | DINNER |
|---|---|---|---|
| **DAY 1** | Sweet Potato Avocado Toast | White Bean Chopped Salad | Salmon with Savory Herbed Quinoa and String Beans |
| **DAY 2** | Sweet Potato Avocado Toast | White Bean Chopped Salad | Salmon with Savory Herbed Quinoa and String Beans |
| **DAY 3** | Sweet Potato Avocado Toast | Salmon with Savory Herbed Quinoa and String Beans | White Bean Chopped Salad |
| **DAY 4** | Sweet Potato Avocado Toast | White Bean Chopped Salad | Salmon with Savory Herbed Quinoa and String Beans |
| **DAY 5** | Sweet Potato Avocado Toast | White Bean Chopped Salad | Salmon with Savory Herbed Quinoa and String Beans |

**Snacks as needed:** Apples and raw almonds
(a serving is 1 apple plus ¼ cup of almonds)

## SHOPPING LIST

### Produce

- Apples (5), for snacking
- Avocados (3)
- Basil (1 bunch)
- Dill (1 bunch)
- Garlic (1 head)
- Green beans (1 pound)
- Lemons (2)
- Lettuce (1 large head)
- Lime (1)
- Onion, red, medium (1)
- Parsley, flat-leaf (2 bunches)
- Radishes (5)
- Scallions (1 bunch)
- Sweet potatoes, large (3)

**Protein**

- Beans, white, 2 (15.5-ounce) cans
- Eggs, large (5)

- Quinoa (1 cup)
- Salmon (1½ pounds)

**Canned/Bottled/Pantry**

- Almonds, raw (1¼ cups), for snacking
- Broth, vegetable (1 quart/32 fluid ounces)
- Cumin, ground
- Honey
- Mustard, Dijon
- Oil, olive

- Oregano, dried
- Peppercorns, black (in a grinder) or ground black pepper
- Salt
- Thyme, dried
- Vinegar, apple cider
- Vinegar, red wine

## EQUIPMENT

- Bowls: 3 large, 2 medium
- Chef's knife and paring knife
- Cutting boards
- Fine-mesh sieve
- Large glass baking dish (9-by-12-inch)
- Large saucepan
- Measuring cups and spoons
- Parchment paper

- Sheet pans, 2 large
- Spatulas
- Storage containers: 5 small, 12 medium, 5 large
- Toaster (or you can toast in the oven)
- Whisk
- Wire cooling rack
- Wooden spoons

## STEP-BY-STEP PREP

1. Follow steps 1 and 2 of the **Salmon with Savory Herbed Quinoa and String Beans** (page 38) to get the fish marinating.

2. Follow steps 1 through 3 of the **Sweet Potato Avocado Toast** (page 35). While the sweet potato and eggs are cooking, complete step 4 and follow the portioning and storage instructions for the avocado mixture in step 5.

3. Set aside the sweet potato slices to cool on a wire rack. You'll reuse the pan for the salmon, and you can keep the oven on at 400°F.

4. Follow step 1 of the **Savory Herbed Quinoa** (page 94). Prepare the green beans for the salmon and quinoa dish (step 4 of the salmon and quinoa recipe). Once the quinoa is cooking, bake the salmon and green beans, following step 5. When the quinoa is cooked, set it aside to cool for 10 minutes.

5. While the quinoa is cooling, follow all the steps for the **White Bean Chopped Salad** (page 37) and follow the storage instructions.

6. Once the salmon is cooked, complete steps 6 through 8 of the salmon and quinoa recipe and follow the storage instructions.

# Sweet Potato Avocado Toast

**DAIRY-FREE • GLUTEN-FREE • NIGHTSHADE-FREE • NUT-FREE • SOY-FREE • VEGETARIAN**
**Makes** 5 servings
**Prep time:** 15 minutes • **Cook time:** 5 minutes

Maximize your vegetable intake first thing in the morning by making "toast" out of sweet potatoes. Feel free to get creative with the toppings, adding in even more veggies if you want to. Prepping avocado ahead of time can be difficult because of avocado's tendency to brown. To keep it fresh over the course of five days, I add water to the top of the mixture.

3 large sweet potatoes, cut lengthwise into ¼-inch-thick slices

5 large eggs

3 avocados, halved and pitted

1 garlic clove, minced

1 teaspoon salt

1 teaspoon freshly ground black pepper

1 teaspoon ground cumin

Juice of 1 lime

5 radishes, finely chopped

1. Preheat the oven to 400°F. Line 1 or 2 large sheet pans with parchment paper.
2. Arrange the sweet potato slices on the sheet pans and bake for 20 minutes, or until tender. They may look like they're not entirely cooked all the way—that's okay; you'll be heating them again later. Transfer them to a wire rack to cool thoroughly.
3. While the potatoes are baking, place the eggs in a pot of water so that they're completely covered. Bring the water to a boil over high heat. When the water boils, remove the pot from the heat, cover, and let stand for 11 minutes. Drain the water and set the eggs aside to cool.
4. Scoop the avocados into a large bowl and mash them lightly with a fork until chunky. Add the garlic, salt, pepper, cumin, lime juice, and radishes. Mix with a wooden spoon until all ingredients are incorporated.

*Continued* ❯

# Sweet Potato Avocado Toast

*Continued*

5. Portion the avocado mixture (about ¼ cup each) into 5 small containers and smooth it with a spoon to eliminate air pockets. Pour 2 tablespoons of cold water on top of the avocado to prevent browning. Store the hard-boiled eggs in a medium container with their shells, or peel them ahead of time (to keep peeled eggs fresh, place a damp paper towel over them and replace it daily). Store the sweet potato slices in a medium container.

✱ **Storage:** Refrigerate everything for up to 4 days. To serve, remove 2 or 3 slices of sweet potato and reheat it in the toaster or oven for 4 to 5 minutes at 400°F. Take out one portion of avocado mixture, pour the water off, stir, then spread it onto the "toast." Take out a hard-boiled egg, slice it, and fan it out on top of the avocado mixture on top of the toast.

✱ **Substitution tip:** To make it vegan, omit the eggs and sprinkle with hemp or pumpkin seeds.

***Per serving (2 toasts):*** *Calories: 364; Total Fat: 23g; Saturated Fat: 5g; Protein: 12g; Total Carbohydrates: 32g; Fiber: 13g; Sugar: 8g; Cholesterol: 186mg*

# White Bean Chopped Salad

**DAIRY-FREE • GLUTEN-FREE • NIGHTSHADE-FREE • NUT-FREE • SOY-FREE • VEGAN**

**Makes** 5 servings
**Prep time:** 20 minutes

A plain lettuce salad is refreshing but not filling. To really enjoy a salad at lunch, you need one that will keep you full and energized all afternoon long. This salad is packed with protein to fuel your body plus fiber and antioxidants for support in calming inflammation.

2 (15.5-ounce) cans
  white beans, drained
  and rinsed
½ medium red
  onion, diced
1 bunch flat-leaf parsley,
  finely chopped
Simple Citrus Vinaigrette
  Dressing (page 86)
5 cups chopped lettuce

1. Place the beans, onion, and parsley in a large bowl.
2. Prepare the vinaigrette as directed. Pour it over the bean mixture. Use a wooden spoon and gently stir to coat the beans. There will be extra dressing at the bottom of the mixture; it will coat the lettuce the mixture is served on later.
3. Portion ¾ cup of the bean mixture into each of 5 medium containers. Portion 1 cup of lettuce greens into 5 separate medium containers.

＊ **Storage:** Store in the refrigerator for up to 5 days. To serve, pour the bean mixture over the lettuce. The dressing from the beans will lightly coat the greens.

＊ **Substitution tip:** There are several types of white beans. Use cannellini, butter beans, great northern, or even white navy beans in this recipe.

*Per serving: Calories: 215; Total Fat: 6g; Saturated Fat: 1g; Protein: 12g; Total Carbohydrates: 31g; Fiber: 8g; Sugar: 1g; Cholesterol: 0mg*

# Salmon with Savory Herbed Quinoa and String Beans

**DAIRY-FREE • GLUTEN-FREE • NIGHTSHADE-FREE • NUT-FREE • SOY-FREE**

**Makes** 5 servings
**Prep time:** 20 minutes • **Cook time:** 20 minutes

This balanced meal, with omega-3-rich salmon, whole-grain quinoa, and delicious string beans, is quick and easy to meal prep so you don't have to worry about what's for dinner all week long. The salmon and beans are roasted on a single sheet pan that you can pop into the oven without a mess.

Fresh Dill Marinade
   (page 87)
1½ pounds skin-on
   salmon fillet
Savory Herbed Quinoa
   (page 94)
1 pound green beans,
   ends snapped off
   (about 3 cups)
1 tablespoon olive oil
Salt
Freshly ground
   black pepper

1. Prepare the dill marinade as directed and transfer it to a 9-by-12-inch glass baking dish.
2. Cut the salmon into five 4- to 5-ounce portions and place it flesh-side down in the marinade for at least 20 minutes.
3. Preheat the oven to 400°F. Line a large sheet pan with parchment paper.
4. While the salmon marinates, start the quinoa recipe (step 1). While the quinoa is cooking, toss the string beans in the oil in a medium bowl and season to taste with salt and pepper.
5. Place the salmon pieces skin-side down along the edges of the sheet pan. Place the beans in the middle of the pan. Bake for 14 to 18 minutes, until the salmon is just cooked through. Baking time will depend on the thickness of the fish.
6. While the salmon is baking, let the quinoa rest, then toss it with the seasonings (step 3), and set it aside.
7. Remove the salmon from the oven to cool.
8. Divide the quinoa evenly into 5 large glass storage containers (about ¾ cup each). Divide the green beans among the containers, placing them on one side of the quinoa. Place a piece of salmon on the other side.

✱ **Storage:** Store in the refrigerator for up to 5 days.

*Per serving: Calories: 411; Total Fat: 17g; Saturated Fat: 3g; Protein: 33g; Total Carbohydrates: 29g; Fiber: 5g; Sugar: 4g; Cholesterol: 75mg*

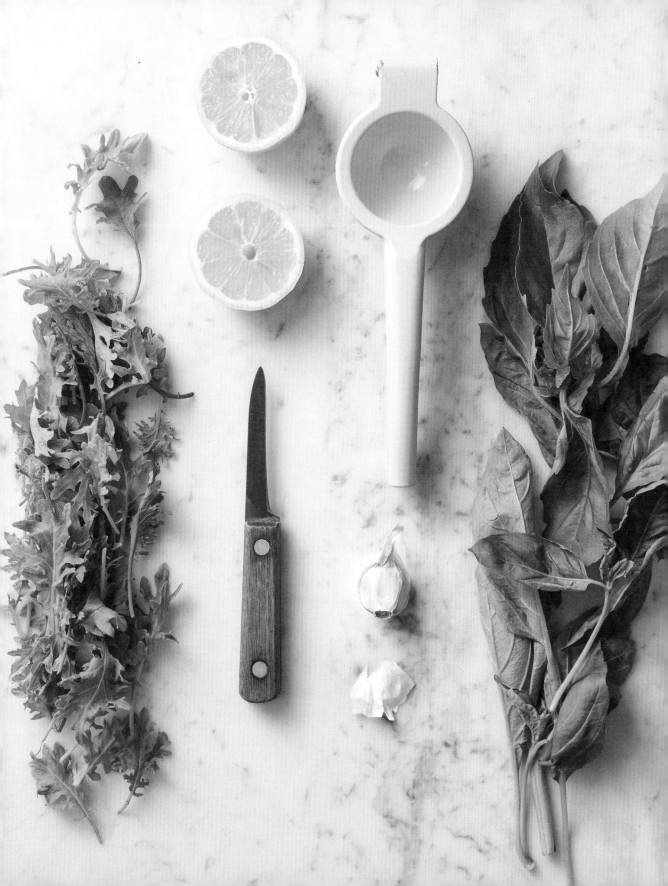

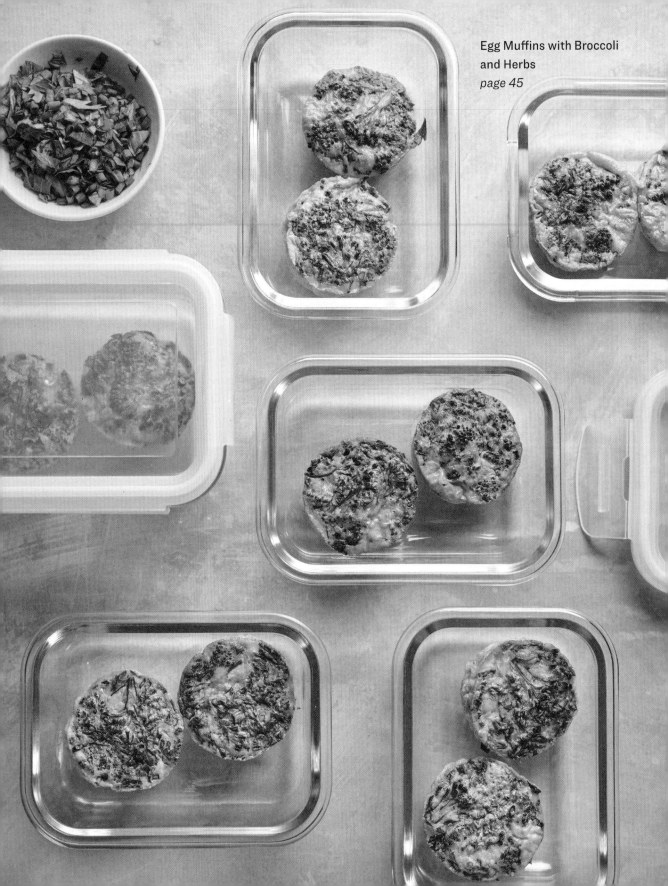

Egg Muffins with Broccoli
and Herbs
*page 45*

# Weeks 3 and 4 Meal Prep

The best way to calm inflammation in your body through nutrition is to eat more fruits and vegetables. There are so many options to choose from—green leafy vegetables like lettuce, spinach, and kale make perfect bases for salads or mix-ins for scrambles. Remember the advice to "eat the rainbow"—colorful vegetables like bell peppers, beans, cucumbers, squash, and sweet potatoes all contain anti-oxidants to support health and calm inflammation. Fruits like melon, berries, apples, pears, stone fruit, tropical fruit, and citrus are all low in calories and rich in nutrients and antioxidants. You already started breaking up with processed foods during Weeks 1 and 2. In Weeks 3 and 4, we'll build on this, looking for more places to fit fruits and vegetables in. Now that you're a little more experienced with meal prep, I'm adding in one additional meal per week to provide more variety.

# Adding More Vegetables to Your Diet Week 3

|  | BREAKFAST | LUNCH | DINNER |
|---|---|---|---|
| **DAY 1** | Egg Muffins with Broccoli and Herbs | Kale Caesar Salad Wraps | Lasagna Roll-Ups |
| **DAY 2** | Egg Muffins with Broccoli and Herbs | Kale Caesar Salad Wraps | Southwestern-Style Stuffed Sweet Potato |
| **DAY 3** | Egg Muffins with Broccoli and Herbs | Southwestern-Style Stuffed Sweet Potato | Lasagna Roll-Ups + Kale Caesar Salad Wraps |
| **DAY 4** | Egg Muffins with Broccoli and Herbs | Kale Caesar Salad Wraps | Lasagna Roll-Ups |
| **DAY 5** | Egg Muffins with Broccoli and Herbs | Lasagna Roll-Ups | Southwestern-Style Stuffed Sweet Potato |

**Snacks as needed:** Edamame in pods (1 serving is 1⅛ cups)

## SHOPPING LIST

### Produce

- Basil (1 bunch)
- Broccoli (1 large head)
- Carrots, medium (2)
- Chives (1 bunch)
- Cilantro (1 bunch)
- Corn kernels (1 cup), or frozen
- Garlic (1 head)
- Kale, lacinato/dinosaur (1 large bunch)

- Lemon (1)
- Lime (1)
- Mushrooms, 1 (8-ounce) container
- Onion, red, medium (1)
- Onion, yellow, medium (1)
- Parsley, flat-leaf (1 bunch)
- Spinach, baby (2 cups)
- Sweet potatoes, medium (3)

### Dairy and Dairy Alternatives

- Mozzarella cheese, shredded, 2 (8-ounce) packages
- Ricotta cheese, 1 (15-ounce) container

### Protein

- Beans, black, 1 (15.5-ounce) can
- Chickpeas, 1 (15.5-ounce) can
- Eggs, large (1 dozen)

### Frozen

- Corn kernels (1 cup), if not using fresh
- Edamame, frozen, unshelled (5¾ cups), for snacking

### Canned/Bottled/Pantry

- Basil, dried
- Capers
- Cumin, ground
- Lasagna noodles, whole wheat (1 box)
- Maple syrup
- Marinara sauce, 2 (25-ounce) jars
- Mustard, Dijon
- Oil, olive
- Oregano, dried
- Peppercorns, black (in a grinder) or ground black pepper
- Salt
- Tahini
- Tortillas, whole wheat, large (3)

## EQUIPMENT

- 12-cup muffin tin
- Aluminum foil
- Bowls: 2 large, 3 medium
- Chef's knife and paring knife
- Colander
- Cutting boards
- Kitchen tongs
- Large glass baking dish (9-by-12-inch)
- Large pot
- Measuring cups and spoons
- Parchment paper
- Resealable bags, for wraps (3)
- Saucepan
- Sheet pan
- Shredder/cheese grater
- Silicone muffin tin liners (if you have them)

- Spatulas
- Storage containers: 8 small (or 12, if using for dressing), 13 medium
- Whisks
- Wooden spoons

## STEP-BY-STEP PREP

1. Follow steps 1 and 2 of the **Southwestern-Style Stuffed Sweet Potato** (page 47). While the sweet potatoes are baking, bring a pot of water to a boil for the noodles for the **Lasagna Roll-Ups** (page 48).

2. Meanwhile, make the filling for the sweet potato recipe (step 3). Portion it into 3 medium containers and refrigerate.

3. When the sweet potatoes are done, set them aside to cool. Leave the oven on but reduce the temperature to 350°F for the lasagna.

4. Add the lasagna noodles to the boiling water and cook (step 2 of the lasagna roll-ups). While the noodles are cooking, make the filling and sauce (steps 3 and 4). While the sauce is simmering, drain the noodles and lay them out to cool on parchment paper (step 2). When the sauce is done, move to steps 5 to 7 to get the lasagna roll-ups in the oven.

5. Complete all the steps of the **Kale Caesar Salad Wraps** (page 46), including storage instructions, and set them in the refrigerator. Complete step 4 of the sweet potato recipe and follow the storage instructions.

6. Assemble the **Egg Muffins with Broccoli and Herbs** (page 45) following steps 1 to 4 and wait for the lasagna to come out of the oven.

7. Once the lasagna is done, set it aside to cool. Put the muffins in the oven (step 5). When the egg muffins are done cooking, set them aside to cool. Portion the lasagna into 6 medium containers, portion the egg muffins into 5 small containers and refrigerate.

# Egg Muffins with Broccoli and Herbs

**DAIRY-FREE • GLUTEN-FREE • NIGHTSHADE-FREE • NUT-FREE • SOY-FREE • VEGETARIAN**

**Makes** 12 egg muffins (6 servings)

**Prep time:** 10 minutes • **Cook time:** 20 minutes

Egg muffins are the perfect delicious vehicle for anti-inflammatory vegetables. They're quick and easy to make, and they're a perfect grab-and-go breakfast or snack (they also freeze well). Eggs tend to stick to muffin tins, so it's worth investing in silicone muffin tin liners.

2 tablespoons olive oil, for greasing (optional)

10 large eggs, beaten

¾ teaspoon salt

¾ teaspoon freshly ground black pepper

2 tablespoons chopped fresh basil

2 tablespoons chopped fresh parsley

2 tablespoons chopped fresh chives

1 cup bite-size pieces broccoli florets

1. Preheat the oven to 350°F. Grease a 12-cup muffin tin with the oil, or use silicone muffin tin liners.
2. In a large bowl, whisk the eggs, salt, and pepper.
3. In a medium bowl, combine the basil, parsley, and chives.
4. Place about 1 tablespoon of chopped broccoli florets in the bottom of each cup, then top it with a small portion of the basil, parsley, and chive mixture. Pour the egg mixture over the broccoli and herbs so that each cup is filled almost to the top.
5. Bake for 20 minutes, then set the muffins aside to cool. Gently scoop them out using a spoon or small spatula, scraping the bottom to ensure nothing sticks to the tin.
6. Portion 2 egg muffins into each of 5 small storage containers.

✳ **Storage:** Store in the refrigerator for up to 5 days, or freeze for future use. To freeze, place the egg cups on a baking sheet and freeze for 2 to 4 hours, then transfer to resealable bags and store for up to 2 months. Thaw in the refrigerator overnight. To serve, microwave for 1 minute.

✳ **Substitution tip:** Feel free to swap in any other herbs or vegetables you enjoy, such as tomato, mushroom, kale, onions, or bell peppers. You can add some cheese or nutritional yeast for extra flavor if desired, based on your dietary plan.

***Per serving (2 egg muffins):*** *Calories: 166; Total Fat: 13g; Saturated Fat: 3g; Protein: 11g; Total Carbohydrates: 2g; Fiber: 1g; Sugar: 1g; Cholesterol: 310mg*

# Kale Caesar Salad Wraps

**DAIRY-FREE • GLUTEN-FREE • NIGHTSHADE-FREE • NUT-FREE • SOY-FREE • VEGAN**
**Makes** 3 wraps (plus 1 extra serving of salad)
**Prep time:** 20 minutes

A veggie wrap is a quick, flavorful, and filling lunch packed with anti-inflammatory ingredients and protein. Sturdy kale leaves make better leftovers than more delicate greens like butter lettuce and spinach. To avoid sogginess, the kale salad is stored separately from the tortillas until you're ready to eat.

1 large bunch lacinato/dinosaur kale

1 (15.5-ounce) can chickpeas, drained and rinsed

2 medium carrots, grated

Zesty Vegan Caesar Dressing (page 88)

3 large whole wheat, corn, or gluten-free tortillas

1. Remove the stems and midribs from the kale leaves, then roughly chop the leaves. Transfer the chopped kale to a large bowl.
2. Add the chickpeas and grated carrots to the bowl.
3. Prepare the Caesar dressing as directed and pour it over the kale mixture. Using your hands or a mixing spoon, stir gently to coat. If you like your kale crispier, skip this step and dress the kale just before serving.
4. Portion the kale Caesar into 4 medium containers (if storing the Caesar dressing separately, portion it into 4 small containers). Roll 3 individual tortillas and wrap them in paper towels. Wrap them again in foil and place in 3 resealable bags.

 * **Storage:** Store in the refrigerator for up to 4 days. To serve the wraps, pour the kale Caesar onto the tortilla, wrap it like a burrito, and enjoy. To make the tortilla softer, microwave it for 15 to 30 seconds before building the wraps.

 * **Reuse tip:** This recipe makes 4 servings but is only served for lunch three times in this prep week, so you'll have extra salad and dressing. Enjoy it as a side to the Lasagna Roll-Ups (page 48) or the Southwestern-Style Stuffed Sweet Potato (page 47). Or make a double batch of dressing to enjoy the following week—it will last in the refrigerator for just under 2 weeks.

*Per serving: Calories: 314; Total Fat: 10g; Saturated Fat: 2g; Protein: 13g; Total Carbohydrates: 46g; Fiber: 10g; Sugar: 9g; Cholesterol: 0mg*

# Southwestern-Style Stuffed Sweet Potato

**DAIRY-FREE • GLUTEN-FREE • NIGHTSHADE-FREE • NUT-FREE • SOY-FREE • VEGAN**

**Makes** 3 servings

**Prep time:** 20 minutes • **Cook time:** 30 minutes

Sweet potatoes are delicious, filling, and packed with vitamins, minerals, and antioxidants. This recipe uses Southwestern-inspired flavors, offering an unexpected combination of vegetables that all help reduce inflammation in the body.

3 medium sweet
   potatoes, well scrubbed

1 tablespoon olive oil

1 teaspoon salt, divided

½ medium red
   onion, diced

1 garlic clove, minced

1 (15.5-ounce) can
   black beans, drained
   and rinsed

1 cup fresh or frozen
   corn kernels

1 teaspoon ground cumin

Juice of 1 lime

½ cup roughly chopped
   fresh cilantro

1. Preheat the oven to 400°F. Line a sheet pan with parchment paper.

2. Halve the sweet potatoes lengthwise. Place them on the sheet pan, cut-side up. Drizzle the oil over the potatoes and rub it in using your fingers. Sprinkle with ½ teaspoon of salt and bake for 30 to 35 minutes, or until the skin is slightly shriveled, the tops are caramelized, and the flesh is tender enough to pierce easily with a fork. Larger potatoes may need more time. Set them aside to cool completely.

3. Meanwhile, to make the filling, in a large bowl, combine the onion, garlic, beans, corn, cumin, and the remaining ½ teaspoon of salt. Stir gently with a wooden spoon, top with the lime juice and cilantro, and toss to coat. Divide the filling mixture into 3 medium containers.

4. Once the potato halves are moderately cool, press a fork into each potato to make an indentation about 1½ inches deep, almost as wide and long as the potato. Take care not to split the sides. Portion the cooled potato halves into 3 small containers.

&ast; **Storage:** To serve, microwave a potato for 1 minute or until it is hot, pour the filling mixture into the indentation, and serve. Refrigerate the potatoes and filling for up to 5 days.

***Per serving:*** *Calories: 335; Total Fat: 6g; Saturated Fat: 1g; Protein: 12g; Total Carbohydrates: 63g; Fiber: 14g; Sugar: 7g; Cholesterol: 0mg*

# Lasagna Roll-Ups

**NUT-FREE • SOY-FREE • VEGETARIAN**
**Makes** 12 roll-ups (6 servings)
**Prep time:** 30 minutes • **Cook time:** 45 minutes

Lasagna has a reputation for being high in calories and fat, but it can also be a wonderful and healthy vehicle for vegetables. This recipe limits the saturated fat by eliminating meat and reducing the amount of cheese, and it boosts the flavor and anti-inflammatory benefits with lots of fresh vegetables and herbs.

12 whole wheat
    lasagna noodles
1 (15-ounce) container
    ricotta cheese
1 large egg
½ cup chopped fresh
    parsley
1 teaspoon dried basil
1 teaspoon dried oregano
½ teaspoon freshly
    ground black pepper
2 cups shredded
    mozzarella
    cheese, divided
2 teaspoons olive oil
½ medium yellow
    onion, diced
1 (8-ounce) container
    mushrooms, sliced
2 garlic cloves, minced
1½ (25-ounce) jars
    marinara sauce, divided
2 cups baby spinach,
    roughly chopped

1. Preheat the oven to 350°F. Bring a large pot of water to a boil over high heat.
2. Add the lasagna noodles to the boiling water and cook for 8 to 10 minutes, until soft. Drain and gently lay the 12 lasagna noodles out flat on a large piece of parchment paper to cool. Use tongs or gloves to avoid burning your fingers.
3. In a medium bowl, combine the ricotta, egg, parsley, basil, oregano, pepper, and ¾ cup of mozzarella. Stir until combined and set it aside.
4. In a saucepan, heat the oil over medium-high heat until warm. Add the onion and sauté for 2 to 3 minutes, or until soft. Add the mushrooms and garlic and cook for 3 to 4 minutes more, until the mushrooms are soft. Add the marinara sauce and spinach. Simmer for 6 minutes and remove from the heat.
5. To assemble the lasagna roll-ups, spread ¼ cup of the ricotta mixture evenly onto each lasagna noodle, leaving a ¼-inch border on each end. On top of the ricotta, spread 2 tablespoons of sauce and 1 tablespoon of mozzarella. Carefully roll up each noodle with the ricotta, sauce, and mozzarella inside.
6. Coat the bottom of a 9-by-12-inch glass baking dish with ½ cup of sauce. Place each lasagna roll, seam-side down, on the sauce in the pan. Top the lasagna rolls with the remaining 2½ cups of sauce and the remaining ½ cup of mozzarella.

7. Cover the baking dish with a large piece of foil and bake for 40 to 45 minutes. Remove the foil and bake it for 5 minutes more, until the mozzarella on top is melted. Set the pan aside to cool.

8. Portion 2 roll-ups each into 6 separate medium containers.

✻ **Storage:** Store in the refrigerator for up to 4 days. To serve, bake in the oven or toaster oven at 350°F for 35 to 40 minutes, until heated through.

✻ **Reuse tip:** This recipe makes 6 servings but is only served four times in this prep week, so you'll have 2 extra servings (4 roll-ups). To freeze extra servings, place cooled roll-ups in airtight containers and store for up to 3 months.

✻ **Substitution tip:** If it suits your health needs, substitute any gluten-free lasagna noodle of your choice. To make this recipe dairy-free, use a nondairy "cheese" substitute and supplement by adding your other favorite vegetables to the sauce.

*Per serving (2 roll-ups): Calories: 488; Total Fat: 19g; Saturated Fat: 10g; Protein: 27g; Total Carbohydrates: 58g; Fiber: 8g; Sugar: 8g; Cholesterol: 89mg*

# Adding More Vegetables to Your Diet Week 4

|  | BREAKFAST | LUNCH | DINNER |
|---|---|---|---|
| **DAY 1** | Blueberry Oatmeal Bake | Chickpea Salad with Creamy Avocado Dressing | Sheet Pan Teriyaki Tofu and Veggies |
| **DAY 2** | Blueberry Oatmeal Bake | Shrimp Pasta with Lemon and Garlic | Sheet Pan Teriyaki Tofu and Veggies |
| **DAY 3** | Blueberry Oatmeal Bake | Chickpea Salad with Creamy Avocado Dressing | Shrimp Pasta with Lemon and Garlic |
| **DAY 4** | Blueberry Oatmeal Bake | Sheet Pan Teriyaki Tofu and Veggies | Shrimp Pasta with Lemon and Garlic |
| **DAY 5** | Blueberry Oatmeal Bake | Chickpea Salad with Creamy Avocado Dressing | Sheet Pan Teriyaki Tofu and Veggies |

**Snacks as needed:** Apples with peanut or almond butter
(1 serving is 1 apple plus 2 tablespoons of nut butter)

## SHOPPING LIST

### Produce

- Apples (5), for snacking
- Avocado (1)
- Blueberries (1 cup), or frozen
- Broccoli (1 head)
- Carrots, medium (4)
- Cauliflower (1 head)
- Celery (2 stalks)
- Cucumber, medium (1)
- Garlic (1 head)
- Ginger (1-inch piece)
- Lemons (2)
- Parsley, curly (1 bunch)
- Spinach, baby (3 cups)

## Protein

- Chickpeas, 2 (15.5-ounce) cans
- Egg, large (1)
- Shrimp, large (¾ pound)
- Tofu, extra-firm, 2 (12-ounce) packages

## Frozen

- Blueberries (1 cup), if not using fresh

## Canned/Bottled/Pantry

- Arrowroot powder or cornstarch
- Bean pasta, such as chickpea, 1 (8-ounce) package
- Cinnamon, ground
- Coconut milk, lite, 1 (13.5-ounce) can
- Honey
- Kalamata olives (4 ounces)
- Maple syrup
- Mustard, Dijon
- Nut butter, peanut or almond
- Oats, old-fashioned rolled (3¼ cups)
- Oil, coconut
- Oil, olive
- Onion powder
- Peppercorns, black (in a grinder) or ground black pepper
- Rice, brown (1 cup)
- Salt
- Sriracha
- Tamari
- Vanilla extract
- Vinegar, apple cider
- Vinegar, rice

## EQUIPMENT

- Bowls: 2 large, 1 medium
- Chef's knife and paring knife
- Colander
- Cutting boards
- Food processor or stand blender
- Glass baking dish (8-by-8-inch)
- Large pot
- Large sheet pan
- Large skillet
- Large whisk
- Medium saucepan
- Measuring cups and spoons
- Parchment paper
- Resealable freezer bag

- Spatulas
- Storage containers: 5 small (or 9, if using for sauce), 8 medium, 7 large
- Wire cooling rack
- Wooden spoons

## STEP-BY-STEP PREP

1. Follow steps 1 to 4 of the **Blueberry Oatmeal Bake** (page 53) and place it in the oven.

2. While the oatmeal bake is in the oven, follow step 1 of **Sheet Pan Teriyaki Tofu and Veggies** (page 55) to prepare the **Basic Brown Rice** (page 93).

3. While the oatmeal bake and brown rice cook, prepare the tofu and vegetables in steps 2 to 4 of the sheet pan tofu. Once the oatmeal bake is finished, set it aside to cool, increase the oven temperature to 425°F, and bake the tofu and veggies per step 5 of the recipe.

4. While the tofu is roasting and the brown rice continues cooking, bring a pot of water to a boil over high heat for the **Shrimp Pasta with Lemon and Garlic** (page 56). Complete steps 1 and 2 for the shrimp pasta. Drain the pasta and broccoli, remove the shrimp from the heat, and allow it to cool.

5. While the sheet pan tofu finishes cooking, follow step 6 of sheet pan tofu to prepare the **Simple Ginger Teriyaki Sauce** (page 90). Follow steps 1 and 2 of the **Chickpea Salad with Creamy Avocado Dressing** (page 54), including storage, and then refrigerate it. Slice and portion the blueberry oat bake into 5 small containers for the week, refrigerate, and place the rest in a freezer bag and freeze for future use.

6. Follow steps 7 and 8 of sheet pan tofu to remove the vegetables from the oven, drizzle them with sauce to taste, and store.

7. Follow steps 3 and 4 of the shrimp pasta and refrigerate.

# Blueberry Oatmeal Bake

**DAIRY-FREE · GLUTEN-FREE · NIGHTSHADE-FREE · NUT-FREE · SOY-FREE · VEGETARIAN**
**Makes** 9 servings
**Prep time:** 5 minutes · **Cook time:** 40 to 45 minutes

Oats bake beautifully in the oven, making a perfect grab-and-go breakfast or snack. This recipe pairs anti-inflammatory oats with antioxidant-rich blueberries and cinnamon. I recommend lite coconut milk for this recipe because it stirs in more easily, but if you need more calories or prefer the richer texture, feel free to use the full-fat version. For more protein, pair with dairy or nondairy yogurt.

½ teaspoon coconut oil

1 large egg

1 (13.5-ounce) can lite coconut milk

¼ cup maple syrup

1 teaspoon pure vanilla extract

½ teaspoon ground cinnamon

¼ teaspoon salt

3¼ cups old-fashioned rolled oats

1 cup fresh or frozen blueberries

1. Preheat the oven to 375°F. Grease an 8-by-8-inch glass baking dish with the coconut oil.
2. In a large bowl, beat the egg. Then add the coconut milk, maple syrup, vanilla, cinnamon, and salt and whisk to combine.
3. To the large bowl, add the oats and blueberries and mix well with a spoon to combine.
4. Spread the oatmeal mixture in the prepared baking dish and bake for 30 to 40 minutes, or until the top is a light, toasty brown. Set on a wire rack to cool.
5. Once cooled, cut the oatmeal bake into 9 squares. Place 5 squares into separate small storage containers. (For the remaining 4 squares, see Reuse tip below.)

＊ **Storage:** Store in the refrigerator for up to 7 days. To serve, enjoy the oat bake cold or microwave it for 30 to 45 seconds.

＊ **Reuse tip:** This recipe makes 9 squares and is only used five times in this prep week. Place the remaining 4 squares in a single layer in a resealable freezer bag; freeze for up to 2 months. Remove one piece at a time from the freezer and thaw overnight in the refrigerator, or microwave to warm.

*Per serving: Calories: 361; Total Fat: 15g; Saturated Fat: 10g; Protein: 11g; Total Carbohydrates: 48g; Fiber: 7g; Sugar: 8g; Cholesterol: 21mg*

# Chickpea Salad with Creamy Avocado Dressing

**DAIRY-FREE • GLUTEN-FREE • NIGHTSHADE-FREE • NUT-FREE • SOY-FREE • VEGAN**
**Makes** 5 servings
**Prep time:** 20 minutes

Hearty chickpeas mixed with a creamy dressing will keep you energized after lunch all week long. This is a high-fiber, protein-packed recipe balanced perfectly with healthy fats plus lots of anti-inflammatory herbs and spices to support your body.

2 (15.5-ounce) cans chickpeas, drained and rinsed
1 medium cucumber, chopped
2 celery stalks, chopped
½ cup chopped kalamata olives
½ cup chopped curly parsley
Creamy Avocado Dressing (page 89)

1. In a large bowl, gently stir together the chickpeas, cucumber, celery, olives, and parsley.
2. Prepare the avocado dressing as directed. Pour the dressing over the chickpea mixture and stir to coat. Divide the dressed salad into 5 medium storage containers.

\* **Storage:** Keep refrigerated for up to 6 days. Serve cold. If following the meal-prep plan, you'll have 2 extra servings (the plan only uses 3 servings).

\* **Substitution tip:** There are several different anti-inflammatory dressings in the Staples chapter (pages 83 to 95). Feel free to swap out the Creamy Avocado Dressing for a different option!

*Per serving:* Calories: 254; Total Fat: 13g; Saturated Fat: 2g; Protein: 8g; Total Carbohydrates: 30g; Fiber: 11g; Sugar: 7g; Cholesterol: 0mg

# Sheet Pan Teriyaki Tofu and Veggies

**DAIRY-FREE • GLUTEN-FREE • NUT-FREE • VEGETARIAN**
**Makes** 4 servings
**Prep time:** 10 minutes • **Cook time:** 30 minutes

Sheet pan meals are a meal-prepper's best friend because you can make a large portion of food on just one sheet and cook it all at once. For this recipe, tofu and veggies are complemented perfectly with a tangy and gingery teriyaki sauce.

Basic Brown Rice
(page 93)
2 (12-ounce) blocks
extra-firm tofu, drained
2 cups cauliflower
florets, chopped into
bite-size pieces
4 medium carrots,
cut into ¼-inch-thick
rounds
1 tablespoon olive oil
½ teaspoon salt
½ teaspoon freshly
ground black pepper
Simple Ginger Teriyaki
Sauce (page 90)

1. Make the brown rice as directed.
2. Preheat the oven to 425°F. Line a large sheet pan with parchment paper.
3. Press the tofu with paper towels to remove excess liquid on the top, bottom, and sides. Slice each block vertically into three slabs, then press them again to remove liquid. Cut the tofu slabs into ½-inch cubes and arrange them on one side of the sheet pan.
4. Place the cauliflower in the middle of the pan and the carrots on the other side, opposite the tofu. Drizzle the tofu and vegetables with the olive oil and sprinkle with the salt and pepper.
5. Bake for 30 minutes, until the tofu is golden brown and the vegetables are tender, flipping them with a spatula halfway through.
6. Meanwhile, make the ginger teriyaki sauce. Remove the brown rice from the heat, fluff, and set it aside to cool.
7. Remove the vegetables and tofu from the oven and set them aside to cool. Drizzle the cooled vegetables and tofu evenly with the ginger teriyaki sauce.
8. Divide the brown rice and tofu plus vegetable combination into 4 large containers. Pour extra sauce directly over the rice or store it in 4 small containers within the large containers to drizzle before serving.

✳ **Storage:** Store in the refrigerator for up to 4 days. To serve, microwave for 1 to 2 minutes.

*Per serving: Calories: 401; Total Fat: 15g; Saturated Fat: 1g; Protein: 23g; Total Carbohydrates: 50g; Fiber: 5g; Sugar: 11g; Cholesterol: 0mg*

# Shrimp Pasta with Lemon and Garlic

**DAIRY-FREE • GLUTEN-FREE • NIGHTSHADE-FREE • NUT-FREE • SOY-FREE**
**Makes** 3 servings
**Prep time:** 10 minutes • **Cook time:** 15 minutes

Yes, you can eat pasta on an anti-inflammatory diet. If you eat gluten, you can swap the bean pasta for whole wheat pasta, which is high in fiber and nutrients, though it's easy nowadays to get bean pastas (mung bean, chickpea, lentil, and others) that are even higher in fiber and protein than grain-based products.

6 ounces bean pasta

1 head broccoli, chopped into florets

3 tablespoons olive oil, divided

¾ pound large shrimp, peeled and deveined

2 garlic cloves, minced

½ teaspoon salt

½ teaspoon freshly ground black pepper

Juice of 1 lemon

3 cups baby spinach

1. Bring a large pot of water to a boil over high heat. Cook the pasta according to package instructions (usually 8 to 10 minutes). Add the broccoli for the final 2 minutes. Drain the pasta and broccoli and set them aside in the same pot they were cooked in.

2. Meanwhile, in a large skillet, heat 2 tablespoons of olive oil over medium heat. Add the shrimp and cook without turning for 5 minutes. Add the garlic, then flip the shrimp to cook on the other side for 3 to 4 minutes, or until cooked through completely and pink in hue. Sprinkle the shrimp with the salt and pepper, add the lemon juice, and cook for 1 minute more.

3. Toss the pasta and broccoli with the remaining 1 tablespoon of olive oil.

4. Place 1 cup of baby spinach into each of 3 medium containers. Divide the broccoli and pasta into 3 large containers. Top each pasta container with a portion of shrimp.

✻ **Storage:** Store in the refrigerator for up to 5 days. To serve, heat the shrimp, pasta, and broccoli mixture in the microwave for 1 to 2 minutes until heated through. Serve over a bed of baby spinach.

✻ **Ingredient tip:** You can save money by buying frozen shrimp, either raw or cooked. Keep them in the freezer and thaw by running under cold water for about 5 minutes before using.

*Per serving:* *Calories: 436; Total Fat: 15g; Saturated Fat: 2g; Protein: 45g; Total Carbohydrates: 32g; Fiber: 16g; Sugar: 3g; Cholesterol: 143mg*

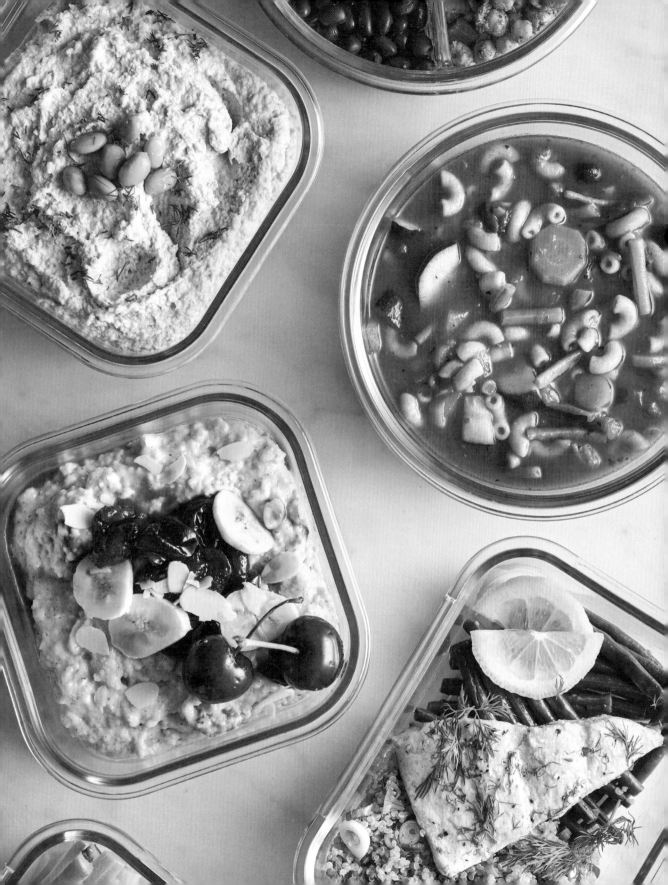

Minestrone Soup with Herbs and
Whole-Grain Pasta

*page 66*

# CHAPTER 5

# Weeks 5 and 6 Meal Prep

For Weeks 5 and 6, we're going to add in more variety at lunch and dinner. That means more anti-inflammatory foods for your body! By now, you're used to keeping whole-food meals on hand each week. Now it's time to add in "super-foods." A superfood is a subjective term that describes a food that is dense in nutrients and serves a functional purpose to health. The focus of this chapter is whole foods that are rich in compounds—including fiber, vitamins, minerals, and antioxidants—that support the body's systems. You'll add more herbs, spices, and colorful antioxidant-rich foods to every meal. As you continue to get better at multitasking in the kitchen on meal-prep day, you'll start rotating in two separate lunches and dinners, giving you the meal plan variety that will keep you sticking with the anti-inflammatory lifestyle long-term.

# Adding in Superfoods Week 5

| | BREAKFAST | LUNCH | DINNER |
|---|---|---|---|
| DAY 1 | Cherry Cocoa Quinoa Breakfast Bowl | Simple Salmon and Romaine Salad with Fresh Vegetables | Garlic-Roasted Tempeh and Veggies |
| DAY 2 | Cherry Cocoa Quinoa Breakfast Bowl | Minestrone Soup with Herbs and Whole-Grain Pasta | Pinto Bean Tacos with Avocado Crema |
| DAY 3 | Cherry Cocoa Quinoa Breakfast Bowl | Simple Salmon and Romaine Salad with Fresh Vegetables | Garlic-Roasted Tempeh and Veggies |
| DAY 4 | Cherry Cocoa Quinoa Breakfast Bowl | Minestrone Soup with Herbs and Whole-Grain Pasta | Pinto Bean Tacos with Avocado Crema |
| DAY 5 | Cherry Cocoa Quinoa Breakfast Bowl | Simple Salmon and Romaine Salad with Fresh Vegetables | Garlic-Roasted Tempeh and Veggies |

**Snacks as needed:** Celery with almond butter and raisins (1 serving is a stalk of celery plus 2 tablespoons of almond butter and ¼ cup of raisins)

## SHOPPING LIST

**Produce**

- Avocado (1)
- Basil (1 bunch)
- Broccoli (1 head)
- Cabbage, green (1 small head)
- Carrots, large (3)
- Celery (1 bunch, includes 5 stalks for snacking)
- Cherries (1 cup), or frozen
- Cilantro (1 bunch)
- Cucumber, medium (1)

- Dill (1 bunch)
- Garlic (1 head)
- Green beans (½ pound)
- Lemons (2)
- Lettuce, romaine (1 head)
- Limes (2)
- Mushrooms, white, 1 (4-ounce) container
- Onion, yellow (1)
- Parsley (1 bunch)

- Scallions (1 bunch)
- Yellow squash (1)
- Zucchini, medium (2)

**Dairy and Dairy Alternatives**

- Soy milk, unsweetened (2 cups)

**Frozen**

- Cherries (1 cup), if not using fresh

**Protein**

- Beans, kidney, 1 (15.5-ounce) can
- Beans, pinto, 1 (15.5-ounce) can
- Salmon (¾ pound)
- Tempeh, 1 (8-ounce) package

**Canned/Bottled/Pantry**

- Almond butter (⅔ cup), for snacking
- Basil, dried
- Broth, vegetable
  (2 quarts/64 fluid ounces)
- Chili powder
- Cocoa powder, unsweetened
- Coconut milk, full-fat, 1 (15-ounce) can
- Cumin, ground
- Garlic powder
- Honey
- Maple syrup
- Mustard, Dijon
- Oil, olive
- Onion powder
- Oregano, dried
- Pasta, elbow or rotini shape, whole wheat or bean (1 cup)
- Peppercorns, black (in a grinder) or ground black pepper
- Quinoa (2 cups)
- Raisins (1¼ cups), for snacking
- Salt
- Thyme, dried
- Tomatoes, diced, 1 (14.5-ounce) can
- Tortillas, corn, soft, 4 (6-inch)
- Vanilla extract
- Vinegar, apple cider
- Vinegar, red wine
- Vinegar, white wine

## EQUIPMENT

- Bowls: 2 large, 3 medium, 1 small
- Chef's knife and paring knife
- Cutting boards
- Fine-mesh sieve

- Foil
- Glass baking dish, 8-by-8-inch
- Kitchen tongs
- Large pot
- Large skillet
- Large whisk
- Measuring cups and spoons
- Parchment paper

- Resealable storage bags, 2
- Saucepan
- Spatulas
- Sheet pans, 2
- Storage containers: 5 small, 12 medium, 12 large
- Wooden spoons

## STEP-BY-STEP PREP

1. Follow steps 1 and 2 of the **Simple Salmon and Romaine Salad with Fresh Vegetables** (page 64) to get the salmon marinating. Skip step 3 and go to step 4 now to make the dressing and salad and store them in the refrigerator.

2. Continue marinating the salmon while you prepare step 1 of the **Garlic-Roasted Tempeh and Veggies** (page 65), which is to marinate the **Garlic-Herb Marinated Tempeh or Tofu** (page 95), steps 2 and 3.

3. While the tempeh marinates, start the **Minestrone Soup with Herbs and Whole-Grain Pasta** (page 66), following steps 1 and 2.

4. While the minestrone soup is coming to a boil or simmering, preheat the oven to 400°F and complete steps 2 to 4 of the garlic-roasted tempeh, cooking the **Savory Herbed Quinoa** (page 94, step 1) and roasting the tempeh and veggies.

5. While the tempeh and veggies are roasting and the quinoa is cooking, move on to step 3 of the minestrone soup. Then start step 1 of the **Cherry Cocoa Quinoa Breakfast Bowl** (page 63) and let it simmer.

6. Remove the tempeh and veggies from the oven and leave the oven on for the salmon, lining the sheet pan (per step 3 of the simple salmon recipe) and baking the salmon (per step 5).

7. Once the salmon is in the oven, complete step 2 of the breakfast bowl. Next, complete step 2 of the herbed quinoa. Then, follow steps 1 to 4 (including storage) of the **Pinto Bean Tacos with Avocado Crema** (page 67).

8. Follow the storage directions for the breakfast bowl; the roasted tempeh, veggies, and herbed quinoa; the cooled minestrone soup; and the baked salmon.

# Cherry Cocoa Quinoa Breakfast Bowl

**DAIRY-FREE • GLUTEN-FREE • NIGHTSHADE-FREE • NUT-FREE • VEGAN**

**Makes** 5 servings

**Prep time:** 10 minutes • **Cook time:** 20 minutes

Quinoa is a high-protein whole grain rich in fiber and antioxidants, offering maximum anti-inflammatory power. It's often served as a savory side dish, but here it's paired with anti-inflammatory cocoa and vibrant cherries to help you start your day. If you don't love chocolate, feel free to add less cocoa, starting with 1 teaspoon and adding more to taste. Or leave the cocoa out completely and enjoy a vanilla-cherry variation instead.

1 cup quinoa, rinsed

2 cups unsweetened
    soy milk

1½ tablespoons
    unsweetened
    cocoa powder

1½ tablespoons
    maple syrup

½ teaspoon pure
    vanilla extract

1 cup fresh or frozen
    cherries, halved
    and pitted

1. In a saucepan, combine the quinoa and soy milk and bring to a boil over medium-high heat. Reduce the heat to medium-low, cover, and simmer for 15 to 20 minutes, until the liquid is absorbed and the quinoa looks fluffy.
2. Transfer the quinoa to a large bowl and add the cocoa, maple syrup, vanilla, and cherries. Mix gently with a wooden spoon and set aside to cool.
3. Divide the cooled quinoa mixture among 5 medium storage containers.

✳ **Storage:** Store in the refrigerator for up to 5 days. Freeze in airtight containers for up to 2 months.

✳ **Ingredient tip:** Especially for this slightly sweet recipe, it's important to rinse the quinoa to eliminate bitterness. Use a fine sieve to rinse the quinoa until the water runs clear.

***Per serving:*** *Calories: 194; Total Fat: 3g; Saturated Fat: 0g; Protein: 8g; Total Carbohydrates: 35g; Fiber: 4g; Sugar: 10g; Cholesterol: 0mg*

# Simple Salmon and Romaine Salad with Fresh Vegetables

**DAIRY-FREE • GLUTEN-FREE • NIGHTSHADE-FREE • NUT-FREE • SOY-FREE**
**Makes** 3 servings
**Prep time:** 30 minutes • **Cook time:** 17 minutes

This easy dish contains many types of anti-inflammatory ingredients, from omega-3s in the salmon to vitamin C and antioxidants in the vegetables and herbs. Salmon, a heart-healthy superfood packed with omega-3s, pairs perfectly with crispy, fresh vegetables and a zesty vinaigrette. You'll enjoy this flavorful, veggie-packed dish all week long.

Fresh Dill Marinade
   (page 87)
¾ pound skin-on
   salmon fillet
Simple Citrus Vinaigrette
   Dressing (page 86)
1 head romaine
   lettuce, chopped
2 large carrots, cut into
   1-inch cubes
2 celery stalks, cut into
   1-inch cubes
1 medium cucumber, cut
   into 1-inch cubes
1 (4-ounce) container
   white mushrooms, cut
   into 1-inch cubes

1. Prepare the dill marinade as directed and transfer it to an 8-by-8-inch glass dish.
2. Cut the salmon into three 4-ounce servings and place it flesh-side down in the marinade. Marinate it for at least 20 minutes while you prep the rest of the ingredients.
3. Preheat the oven to 400°F. Line a large sheet pan with parchment paper.
4. While the oven heats, prepare the vinaigrette dressing as directed. Store the dressing in 3 small containers. In a large bowl, toss together the lettuce, carrots, celery, cucumber, and mushrooms. Store the salad in 3 large containers.
5. Remove the salmon from the marinade and place it skin-down on the sheet pan. Bake for 13 to 17 minutes, until the salmon is just cooked through (the baking time will vary based on the thickness of the fish).
6. Remove the salmon from the oven and set it aside to cool. Store the salmon in 3 medium containers.

   ✱ **Storage:** Store in the refrigerator for up to 5 days. To serve, dress the salad, microwave the salmon for 1 minute (or serve cold), and serve it on top of the salad.

   *Per serving: Calories: 342; Total Fat: 15g; Saturated Fat: 3g; Protein: 35g; Total Carbohydrates: 15g; Fiber: 7g; Sugar: 6g; Cholesterol: 83mg*

# Garlic-Roasted Tempeh and Veggies

**DAIRY-FREE • GLUTEN-FREE • NIGHTSHADE-FREE • NUT-FREE • VEGAN**
**Makes** 3 servings
**Prep time:** 15 minutes • **Cook time:** 20 minutes

This simple sheet pan meal is a hands-off meal-prep staple that allows you to focus on preparing other recipes while it cooks. The superfood tempeh is coated with savory garlic, and the hearty, anti-inflammatory superfood vegetables—broccoli, zucchini, and yellow squash—bake well and will hold up as leftovers all week.

Garlic-Herb Marinated
  Tempeh or Tofu
  (page 95)
1½ cups Savory Herbed
  Quinoa (page 94)
2 cups broccoli florets
1 medium zucchini,
  quartered lengthwise
  and sliced
1 yellow squash,
  quartered lengthwise
  and sliced

1. Prepare the tempeh as directed and set it aside to marinate (steps 2 and 3).
2. Start cooking the quinoa (step 1 only).
3. While the quinoa cooks, preheat the oven to 400°F. Line a sheet pan with parchment paper.
4. Place the broccoli, zucchini, and yellow squash on one side of the sheet pan. Remove the tempeh from its marinade with tongs and place it on the other side of the sheet pan. Drizzle the tempeh and vegetables evenly with the extra marinade. Bake for 15 to 20 minutes, flipping with a spatula halfway through, until the vegetables have softened.
5. Remove the quinoa from the heat and follow steps 2 and 3 of the recipe.
6. In 3 separate large containers, portion out the quinoa on one side, the roasted vegetables in the middle, and the tempeh on the other side.

✽ **Storage:** Store in the refrigerator for up to 4 days. To serve, microwave for 1 to 2 minutes or until heated through.

✽ **Substitution tip:** You can use tofu instead of tempeh to switch things up. If you want more protein in this dish, feel free to make two batches instead of just one.

*Per serving: Calories: 428; Total Fat: 23g; Saturated Fat: 4g; Protein: 21g; Total Carbohydrates: 38g; Fiber: 5g; Sugar: 3g; Cholesterol: 0mg*

# Minestrone Soup with Herbs and Whole-Grain Pasta

**DAIRY-FREE • GLUTEN-FREE • NUT-FREE • SOY-FREE • VEGAN**
**Makes** 6 servings
**Prep time:** 10 minutes • **Cook time:** 45 minutes

Minestrone is a filling and well-balanced Italian-inspired soup with fiber- and protein-rich beans, a variety of antioxidant-packed veggies, and whole-grain pasta. As minestrone is traditionally a tomato-based soup, this recipe is not nightshade-free (though, if you're not sensitive to nightshades, they can be very anti-inflammatory).

2 tablespoons olive oil
½ yellow onion, diced
1 large carrot, cut into thin rounds
1 cup green beans, trimmed and cut into thirds
1 medium zucchini, halved lengthwise and cut crosswise into ¼-inch half-moons
2 garlic cloves, minced
1 teaspoon dried basil
1 teaspoon dried oregano
1 teaspoon salt
1 teaspoon freshly ground black pepper
1 (14.5-ounce) can diced tomatoes
4 cups vegetable broth
1 (15.5-ounce) can kidney beans, drained and rinsed
1 cup whole wheat or bean rotini or elbow pasta

1. In a large pot, warm the olive oil over medium-high heat. Add the onion, carrot, green beans, and zucchini and cook for 10 to 12 minutes, or until the onions are translucent and the vegetables soften. Add the garlic, basil, oregano, salt, and pepper and cook for another 1 to 2 minutes, stirring frequently.

2. Add the tomatoes and broth. Increase the heat to medium-high and bring the soup to a boil. Then cover, reduce the heat to medium-low, and let simmer for 15 minutes.

3. Add the canned beans and uncooked pasta and cook, uncovered, for 11 to 15 minutes more, until the pasta is tender. Allow to cool before storing.

4. Portion the soup into 6 large containers.

❋ **Storage:** This recipe yields 6 servings, but the meal plan only uses two. Freeze the other 4 servings for future weeks or eat as a snack or side. Store in the refrigerator for up to 5 days, or freeze for up to 2 months.

❋ **Substitution tip:** This soup also tastes great prepared spicy—add ½ teaspoon of red pepper flakes if you enjoy spicy food. Other herbs, like fresh basil, fresh dill, thyme, or a bay leaf (removed when the soup is finished) also fit well in this recipe and provide antioxidants.

***Per serving:*** *Calories: 161; Total Fat: 5g; Saturated Fat: 1g; Protein: 6g; Total Carbohydrates: 25g; Fiber: 6g; Sugar: 5g; Cholesterol: 0mg*

# Pinto Bean Tacos with Avocado Crema

**DAIRY-FREE • GLUTEN-FREE • NUT-FREE • SOY-FREE • VEGAN**

**Makes** 4 tacos (2 servings)

**Prep time:** 10 minutes • **Cook time:** 10 minutes

Pinto beans are full of fiber and protein and are easy to build a meal around for lunch or dinner. Cooked here with savory onion, garlic, and an anti-inflammatory spice blend, they become the plant-based star of the show. This recipe is garnished with additional super-foods, like cilantro, avocado, and lime.

1 tablespoon olive oil

½ yellow onion, diced

1 garlic clove, minced

1 (15.5-ounce) can
   pinto beans, drained
   and rinsed

2 tablespoons
   Anti-Inflammatory
   Multiuse Spice Blend
   (page 84)

Juice of 1 lime

½ cup Avocado Crema
   (page 91)

½ cup shredded
   green cabbage

½ cup chopped
   fresh cilantro

4 (6-inch) corn tortillas

1. In a large skillet, warm the olive oil over medium-high heat. Add the onion and cook for 2 to 4 minutes, or until softened.

2. Add the garlic and cook for 1 minute more. Add the pinto beans, spice blend, and lime juice. Stir well for 1 to 2 minutes, until the mixture is heated through and all the ingredients are incorporated. Let cool, then divide the pinto beans between 2 medium containers.

3. Prepare the avocado crema as directed. Divide between 2 small storage containers.

4. Divide the cabbage between 2 medium containers and top with the cilantro. Roll the tortillas in 2 sets of 2, then wrap in paper towel and then foil. Twist the ends and store in airtight bags.

\* **Storage:** Refrigerate all components for up to 5 days. To serve, microwave the tortillas for 10 to 20 seconds to warm. Microwave the pinto bean mixture for 30 to 60 seconds until heated through and pour onto tortillas. Garnish the tacos with cabbage, cilantro, and avocado crema.

\* **Reuse tip:** Tortillas freeze well, so freeze the rest of the package of tortillas to keep fresh for next time.

*Per serving (2 tacos):* Calories: 492; Total Fat: 20g; Saturated Fat: 5g; Protein: 17g; Total Carbohydrates: 68g; Fiber: 20g; Sugar: 5g; Cholesterol: 0mg

# Adding in Superfoods Week 6

|  | BREAKFAST | LUNCH | DINNER |
|---|---|---|---|
| **DAY 1** | Ginger-Berry Granola | Citrus, Beet, and Chickpea Salad with Fresh Herbs | Butternut Squash, Spinach, and White Bean Enchiladas |
| **DAY 2** | Ginger-Berry Granola | Vegetable Fried Cauliflower Rice | Lentil Dal with Brown Rice |
| **DAY 3** | Ginger-Berry Granola | Citrus, Beet, and Chickpea Salad with Fresh Herbs | Butternut Squash, Spinach, and White Bean Enchiladas |
| **DAY 4** | Ginger-Berry Granola | Vegetable Fried Cauliflower Rice | Lentil Dal with Brown Rice |
| **DAY 5** | Ginger-Berry Granola | Lentil Dal with Brown Rice | Butternut Squash, Spinach, and White Bean Enchiladas |

**Snacks as needed:** 1 batch Banana Energy Cookies (page 149)

## SHOPPING LIST

**Produce**

- Bananas (2)
- Basil (1 bunch)
- Beets, red, medium (2)
- Blueberries (2 cups), or frozen
- Butternut squash (1 small) or 1 bag chopped butternut squash
- Carrots (2)
- Cauliflower (1 head) or 12 ounces frozen riced cauliflower
- Cilantro (1 bunch)
- Dill (1 bunch)
- Garlic (1 head)
- Ginger (3-inch piece)
- Lettuce (1 small head)
- Onion, red, small (1)
- Onion, yellow, medium (1)
- Oranges (2)

- Peas (1 cup), or frozen
- Potatoes, golden, medium (2)

- Scallions (1 bunch)
- Spinach, baby (5 cups)

## Dairy and Dairy Alternatives

- Jack cheese, shredded, 1 (8-ounce) package

- Optional: Soy milk or yogurt, for serving with granola

## Frozen

- Blueberries (2 cups), if not using fresh
- Cauliflower, riced, 1 (12-ounce) package, if not using fresh

- Peas (1 cup), if not using fresh

## Protein

- Beans, white, 1 (15.5-ounce) can
- Chickpeas, 1 (15.5-ounce) can

- Eggs, large (2)
- Tofu, firm, 1 (15-ounce) package

## Canned/Bottled/Pantry

- Almonds, slivered (1 cup)
- Basil, dried
- Broth, vegetable (¼ cup)
- Chia seeds (2 tablespoons)
- Chili powder
- Coriander, ground
- Cumin, ground
- Flour, whole wheat or gluten-free (¼ cup)
- Garlic powder
- Honey
- Lentils, brown (½ cup)
- Maple syrup
- Mustard, Dijon
- Oats, old-fashioned rolled (4 cups)
- Oil, canola

- Oil, coconut
- Oil, olive
- Oil, sesame
- Onion powder
- Oregano, dried
- Peppercorns, black (in a grinder) or ground black pepper
- Rice, brown (1 cup)
- Salt
- Tamari
- Thyme, dried
- Tomato sauce, 1 (28-ounce) can
- Tortillas, whole wheat, 8 (8-inch)
- Turmeric, ground
- Vanilla extract
- Vinegar, apple cider

- Vinegar, rice
- Vinegar, white wine

- Optional: ½ cup mix-ins for Banana Energy Cookies (page 149), such as walnuts, chocolate chips, dried cranberries, or ground cinnamon

## EQUIPMENT

- Bowls: 2 large, 4 medium, 1 small
- Cheese grater
- Chef's knife and paring knife
- Colander
- Cutting boards
- Foil
- Large glass baking dish (9-by-12-inch)
- Large pot

- Large skillet
- Large whisk
- Measuring cups and spoons
- Parchment paper
- Saucepan
- Sheet pan
- Spatulas
- Storage containers: 16 medium, 8 large
- Wooden spoons

## STEP-BY-STEP PREP

1. Follow steps 1 and 2 of the **Citrus, Beet, and Chickpea Salad with Fresh Herbs** (page 73).

2. While the beets are baking, follow steps 1 to 3 of the **Homemade Enchilada Sauce** (page 92) for step 1 of the **Butternut Squash, Spinach, and White Bean Enchiladas** (page 76) and transfer the sauce to a medium bowl.

3. Use the pot from the enchilada sauce to make the **Basic Brown Rice** (page 93, steps 1 and 2) for step 1 of the **Lentil Dal with Brown Rice** (page 78).

4. While the beets are baking and the rice is cooking, complete steps 3 and 4 of the beet and chickpea salad. Then, start step 1 of the **Vegetable Fried Cauliflower Rice** (page 74) by preparing the **Garlic-Herb Marinated Tempeh or Tofu** (page 95, steps 2 and 3) and setting it aside to marinate.

5. Once the beets are done, remove them from the oven and set them aside to cool. Reduce the oven temperature to 325°F and follow steps 1 to 4 of the **Ginger-Berry Granola** (page 72).

6. While the granola is baking, complete steps 3 to 7 of the enchiladas—though don't change the oven temperature yet. Complete steps 5 and 6 of the beet and chickpea salad and refrigerate.

7. Once the granola is cooked, remove it from the oven and set it aside to cool. Make the **Banana Energy Cookies** (page 149) by following steps 1 to 4.

8. When the cookies are done baking, remove them from the oven and set them aside to cool. Increase the oven temperature to 400°F and bake the enchiladas (step 8).

9. While the enchiladas are baking, cook the lentils for the lentil dal, completing steps 2 to 5 (including storage).

10. Once the enchiladas are done cooking, remove them from the oven and set them aside to cool. Complete steps 1 and 4 of the marinated tofu, baking at 400°F.

11. While the tofu bakes, complete steps 2 to 7 of the fried cauliflower rice and set it aside to cool. Then complete step 8, removing the marinated tofu from the oven and setting it aside to cool. Portion the cauliflower rice and tofu into storage containers, as directed.

12. Portion the cooled granola into 5 medium containers and store them in the refrigerator. Place the cooled cookies in a large storage container and store at room temperature.

# Ginger-Berry Granola

**DAIRY-FREE · GLUTEN-FREE · NIGHTSHADE-FREE · SOY-FREE · VEGETARIAN**
**Makes** 6 servings
**Prep time:** 10 minutes · **Cook time:** 30 minutes

This easy, delicious, homemade granola is low in added sugar and oil but is packed with healthy, anti-inflammatory superfoods like chia seeds, ginger, blueberries, and oats. Serve it with soy milk or yogurt for extra protein.

3 cups old-fashioned rolled oats

1 cup slivered almonds

2 tablespoons chia seeds

¼ teaspoon salt

1-inch piece fresh ginger, grated

½ cup honey

⅓ cup olive oil

1 teaspoon pure vanilla extract

2 cups fresh or frozen blueberries

Optional: Soy milk or yogurt, for serving

1. Preheat the oven to 325°F. Line a large sheet pan with parchment paper.
2. In a large bowl, combine the oats, almonds, chia seeds, salt, and ginger with a wooden spoon.
3. In a medium bowl, whisk together the honey, olive oil, and vanilla. Pour the honey mixture over the oat mixture and stir well to combine.
4. Mix the blueberries into the oats, then spread the granola on the prepared sheet pan. Bake for 30 to 40 minutes, stirring halfway through to ensure it cooks evenly. Watch the corners because they tend to get brown. Cool before storing.
5. Divide the granola into 6 medium containers.

∗ **Storage:** Store in the refrigerator for up to 7 days. Granola freezes well, and this recipe makes 6 servings but is only used five times in this week's meal plan. Freeze extra granola for up to 3 months.

∗ **Substitution tip:** For more antioxidants, add even more berries! Try using fresh or frozen mixed berries. In place of almonds, feel free to use pecans, hazelnuts, walnuts, or even pumpkin or sunflower seeds or coconut. To make this recipe vegan, use maple syrup instead of honey.

*Per serving: Calories: 502; Total Fat: 24g; Saturated Fat: 3g; Protein: 11g; Total Carbohydrates: 65g; Fiber: 10g; Sugar: 28g; Cholesterol: 0mg*

# Citrus, Beet, and Chickpea Salad with Fresh Herbs

**DAIRY-FREE • GLUTEN-FREE • NIGHTSHADE-FREE • NUT-FREE • SOY-FREE • VEGAN**
**Makes** 2 servings
**Prep time:** 20 minutes • **Cook time:** 1 hour

Enjoy lunchtime with a hearty superfood salad that combines anti-inflammatory vegetables, fruit, and protein-packed chickpeas. Flavors pop in this recipe—bright citrus and earthy beets provide a striking flavor balance. This highly portable salad will keep your energy high throughout the afternoon.

2 medium red beets

2 medium oranges, peeled, segmented, and segments cut in half

1 (15.5-ounce) can chickpeas, drained and rinsed

¼ cup apple cider vinegar

¼ cup olive oil

½ teaspoon Dijon mustard

3 tablespoons coarsely chopped fresh basil

3 tablespoons coarsely chopped fresh dill

½ teaspoon maple syrup

½ teaspoon salt

½ teaspoon freshly ground black pepper

2 cups chopped lettuce

1. Preheat the oven to 425°F.
2. Wrap the beets in foil and roast them directly on the oven rack for 40 minutes to 1 hour, until they can easily be pierced with a knife.
3. While the beets are cooking, place the orange slices in a medium bowl. Add the chickpeas and set aside.
4. In a separate medium bowl, whisk together the vinegar, oil, mustard, basil, dill, maple syrup, salt, and pepper. Pour it over the orange and chickpea mixture and mix gently to coat.
5. Once the beets are cooked, remove them from the oven and set them aside to cool. Once they're safe to handle with bare (or gloved) hands, use your thumbs to gently peel off the outer skin. Cut them into 1-inch cubes, add them to the bowl with the oranges, chickpeas, and dressing, and stir gently to coat.
6. Divide the lettuce into 2 large containers (when it comes time to serve, you will add the other ingredients to the lettuce, which is why you need a large container). Divide the orange, beet, and chickpea mixture into 2 medium containers.

* **Storage:** Store in the refrigerator for up to 4 days. To serve, pour the orange, beet, and chickpea mixture over the lettuce and serve cold.

*Per serving: Calories: 564; Total Fat: 31g; Saturated Fat: 4g; Protein: 14g; Total Carbohydrates: 62g; Fiber: 15g; Sugar: 25g; Cholesterol: 0mg*

# Vegetable Fried Cauliflower Rice

**DAIRY-FREE • GLUTEN-FREE • NIGHTSHADE-FREE • NUT-FREE • VEGETARIAN**
**Makes** 4 servings
**Prep time:** 15 minutes • **Cook time:** 15 minutes

Cauliflower rice is the key to an anti-inflammatory, superfood stir-fry. Perfectly balanced with protein from nutrient-dense tofu, this satisfying and flavorful dish is packed with vegetables, herbs, and spices. In this recipe, you'll make a simple homemade version of stir-fry sauce—an easy way to cut out added sugars and preservatives found in store-bought options. You can grate your own cauliflower or, to save time, purchase a frozen "riced" variety.

Garlic-Herb Marinated
  Tempeh or Tofu
  (page 95)
1 head cauliflower, or
  1 (12-ounce) package
  frozen riced cauliflower
3 tablespoons tamari
½ teaspoon honey
1 teaspoon rice vinegar
1 tablespoon coconut oil
1 carrot, sliced into
  thin rounds
2 garlic cloves, minced
1 tablespoon finely
  chopped fresh ginger
1 tablespoon water
1 cup green peas, fresh
  or frozen
1 tablespoon sesame oil
2 large eggs, beaten
2 scallions, minced

1. Preheat the oven and marinate the tofu as directed (steps 1 to 3).
2. While the tofu marinates, cut the cauliflower into quarters, remove the stem and core, then "rice" it using the largest side of a box grater (once grated, pieces should be the size of grains of rice). If you're using a bag of frozen riced cauliflower, open the bag and set it aside.
3. In a small bowl, whisk together the tamari, honey, and vinegar. Set it aside.
4. Move the tofu to the oven (step 4 of the marinated tofu recipe).
5. While the tofu bakes, in a large skillet, heat the coconut oil over medium heat. Add the carrot, garlic, and ginger and cook, stirring often, for 3 to 4 minutes, or until the carrot softens and the garlic is fragrant. If the mixture is dry, add water 1 teaspoon at a time so the carrots can continue cooking.
6. Add the riced cauliflower and peas to the pan. Stir frequently to stir-fry the cauliflower until it softens and then begins to crisp, 4 to 7 minutes.
7. Make a well in the middle of the cauliflower mixture and add the sesame oil. Heat the oil for 30 seconds, then pour the eggs on top of the oil. Stir the eggs constantly to scramble them, for 2 to 3 minutes, until fully cooked. Stir the cooked eggs into the mixture. Add the tamari, honey, and vinegar mixture to the skillet and stir to coat.

8. Remove the tofu from the oven and set it aside to cool.
9. Divide the cauliflower rice evenly into 2 medium storage containers and top with the tofu and scallions. (See Reuse tip for the remaining portions.)

✳ **Storage:** Store in the refrigerator. To serve, microwave for 1 to 2 minutes or until warmed through.

✳ **Reuse tip:** This recipe makes 4 servings but is only called for two times in the meal prep. So portion leftovers into 2 additional containers or freeze for up to 2 months. Thaw overnight in the refrigerator before reheating.

✳ **Cooking tip:** If you have a food processor, skip the grating by putting large chunks of cauliflower in the food processor and pulsing to "rice" it. If grating by hand, avoid the mess by setting the grater inside a large bowl or glass baking dish.

*Per serving:* Calories: 318; Total Fat: 23g; Saturated Fat: 7g; Protein: 18g; Total Carbohydrates: 16g; Fiber: 3g; Sugar: 3g; Cholesterol: 93mg

# Butternut Squash, Spinach, and White Bean Enchiladas

**NUT-FREE • SOY-FREE • VEGETARIAN**
**Makes** 8 enchiladas (4 servings)
**Prep time:** 20 minutes • **Cook time:** 40 minutes

Enchiladas are often associated with comfort food, but they can be made healthy when prepared with anti-inflammatory superfoods like squash, spinach, and beans. This recipe uses white beans, but you can swap in any bean you like. Making your own sauce is easy, quick, and allows you to choose ingredients to suit your health and your flavor preferences.

Homemade Enchilada
  Sauce, divided
  (page 92)
2 tablespoons olive oil
1 small red onion, diced
2 garlic cloves, minced
1 cup cubed butternut
  squash
3 tablespoons water
1 teaspoon ground cumin
½ teaspoon salt
½ teaspoon freshly
  ground black pepper
5 cups baby spinach
1 (15.5-ounce) can
  white beans, drained
  and rinsed
1 cup shredded Jack
  cheese, divided
8 (8-inch) whole wheat
  or corn tortillas
½ cup chopped
  fresh cilantro

1. Prepare the enchilada sauce as directed.
2. Preheat the oven to 400°F.
3. Pour ⅓ cup of enchilada sauce into a 9-by-12-inch glass baking dish to cover the bottom evenly in a thin layer.
4. In a large skillet, heat the oil over medium heat. Add the onion, garlic, and butternut squash, stirring occasionally for 5 to 7 minutes, or until the vegetables soften. If the mixture is starting to caramelize, add water a tablespoon at a time to prevent sticking.
5. Add the cumin, stir to incorporate, then cover and let the mixture continue to cook, stirring occasionally, for 3 to 4 minutes more, or until the squash can be pierced easily with a fork.
6. When the squash is soft, sprinkle the mixture with the salt and pepper, then add the spinach. Cook, stirring occasionally, for 3 to 5 minutes, or until the spinach is wilted and incorporated. Remove from the heat and transfer the filling to a large bowl. Add the beans and ½ cup of cheese and stir to incorporate.
7. Place one tortilla at a time on a cutting board or clean surface. Pour ½ cup of filling mixture into the middle, then top with ¼ cup of enchilada sauce. Carefully fold the tortilla around the filling so that the edges overlap slightly. Place the filled tortilla seam-side down into the baking dish. Repeat with the remaining tortillas, setting them in a row to fill the dish completely.

8. Pour the remaining enchilada sauce on top of the prepared enchiladas and sprinkle the remaining ½ cup of cheese evenly over the top. Bake for 20 to 30 minutes, or until the enchiladas are bubbling hot and golden brown on the edges. Remove from the oven and let cool. Sprinkle with the cilantro.
9. Place 2 enchiladas in each of 4 large storage containers (see Reuse tip).

✳ **Storage:** Store in the refrigerator for up to 6 days. To serve, microwave the enchiladas for 1 to 2 minutes or until heated through.

✳ **Reuse tip:** This makes 4 servings but it's only called for three times in the meal prep this week. So if you'd like, you can freeze the other container for up to 2 months, or refrigerate it for up to 6 days.

✳ **Substitution tip:** This recipe can easily be made gluten-free by using corn tortillas and gluten-free flour blend in the enchilada sauce. To make it dairy-free, use a nondairy cheese. This recipe can't be made nightshade-free because the sauce is tomato-based, and the spice blend uses chili powder.

*Per serving (2 enchiladas):* Calories: 601; Total Fat: 33g; Saturated Fat: 8g; Protein: 21g; Total Carbohydrates: 64g; Fiber: 15g; Sugar: 10g; Cholesterol: 25mg

# Lentil Dal with Brown Rice

**DAIRY-FREE · GLUTEN-FREE · NIGHTSHADE-FREE · NUT-FREE · SOY-FREE · VEGAN**
**Makes** 3 servings
**Prep time:** 15 minutes · **Cook time:** 30 minutes

Dal, sometimes spelled *dhal*, is a widely varying lentil-based dish with origins in Indian cuisine. This simple, one-pot dal is full of anti-inflammatory ingredients and spices, like coriander, turmeric, and cumin. Lentils make great leftovers, as they keep well in the refrigerator and freezer.

1 cup Basic Brown Rice
   (page 93)
2 tablespoons coconut oil
1 medium yellow
   onion, diced
2 garlic cloves, minced
1-inch piece fresh
   ginger, grated
2 teaspoons ground
   coriander
1 teaspoon ground cumin
1 teaspoon ground
   turmeric
4 cups water, plus
   2 tablespoons
2 golden potatoes, diced
1 carrot, cut into
   thin rounds
½ cup brown lentils
1 teaspoon salt
½ teaspoon freshly
   ground black pepper

1. Make the brown rice.
2. While the rice cooks, in a large pot, heat the coconut oil over medium heat. Add the onion and cook for 3 to 4 minutes, or until softened. Add the garlic, ginger, coriander, cumin, and turmeric and cook for 1 minute, stirring frequently, until the spices are incorporated and fragrant. Add 1 tablespoon of water and gently scrape the bottom of the pot where spices and vegetables are sticking.
3. Add the potatoes and carrot and cook for 2 minutes, stirring frequently to coat the vegetables with spices. If the vegetables are sticking to the bottom of the pan, add another tablespoon of water and scrape up the stuck bits.
4. Add the lentils, salt, pepper, and remaining 4 cups of water. Increase the heat to medium-high and bring the mixture to a boil, then reduce the heat to low and simmer for 20 to 25 minutes, or until the lentils are soft and the potatoes are cooked through.
5. Remove the dal and brown rice from the heat. When cooled, divide the rice into 3 medium containers, then top with dal.

✳ **Storage:** Store in the refrigerator for up to 5 days To serve, microwave for 1 to 2 minutes, until heated through. Freeze leftovers for up to 2 months.

***Per serving:*** *Calories: 436; Total Fat: 11g; Saturated Fat: 8g; Protein: 15g; Total Carbohydrates: 78g; Fiber: 9g; Sugar: 4g; Cholesterol: 0mg*

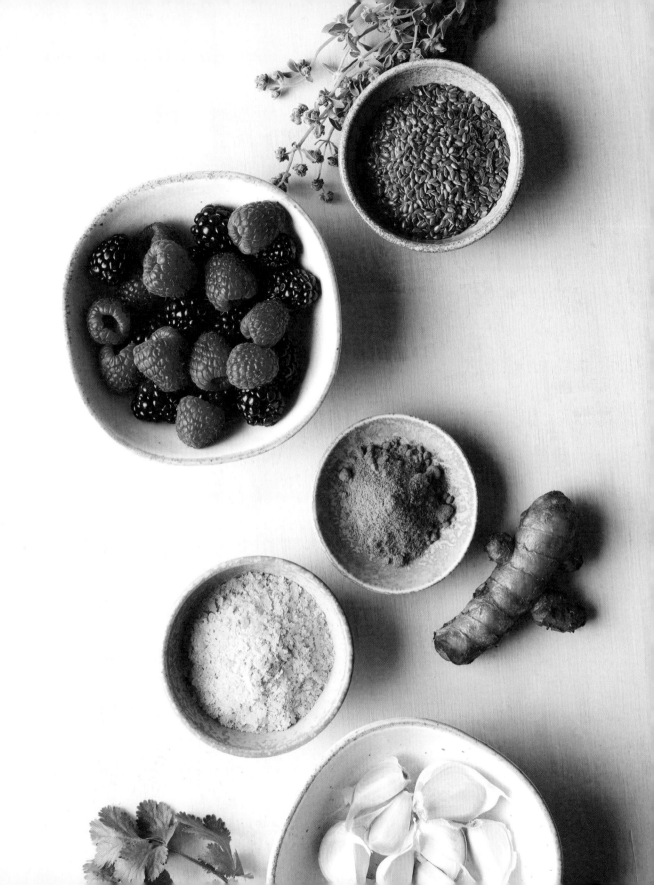

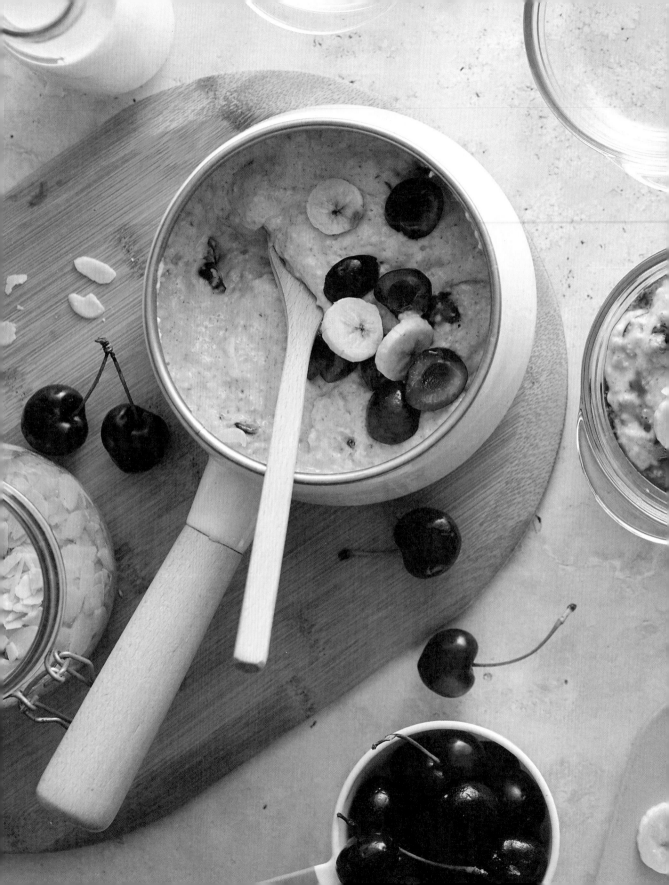

# PART THREE

# More Recipes to Prep

||||||||||||||||||

Savory Herbed Quinoa

*page 94*

CHAPTER

# 6

# Staples

# Anti-Inflammatory Multiuse Spice Blend

**DAIRY-FREE • GLUTEN-FREE • NUT-FREE • SOY-FREE • VEGAN**

**Makes** ⅓ cup
**Prep time:** 5 minutes

A staple spice blend is key for any anti-inflammatory diet. Blends you buy in the store may include fillers and artificial flavor enhancers. Instead, make your own in a matter of minutes by combining several anti-inflammatory spices. Use this mix to make endless recipes flavorful.

2½ teaspoons
   chili powder

2½ teaspoons
   garlic powder

2 teaspoons
   ground cumin

1½ teaspoons
   onion powder

2 teaspoons
   dried oregano

1 teaspoon dried basil

1 teaspoon salt

1 teaspoon freshly ground
   black pepper

In a small bowl, combine the chili powder, garlic powder, cumin, onion powder, oregano, basil, salt, and pepper.

❋ **Storage:** Store in a small container for up to 1 year.

❋ **Substitution tip:** Make a spicier version of this blend by adding an extra teaspoon of chili powder or red pepper flakes. Feel free to double or triple the recipe so you always have plenty on hand.

***Per serving (1 tablespoon):*** *Calories: 17; Total Fat: 0g; Saturated Fat: 0g; Protein: 1g; Total Carbohydrates: 3g; Fiber: 1g; Sugar: 0g; Cholesterol: 0mg*

# Honey-Lime Vinaigrette with Fresh Herbs

**DAIRY-FREE • GLUTEN-FREE • NIGHTSHADE-FREE • NUT-FREE • SOY-FREE • VEGETARIAN**
**Makes** 1 cup
**Prep time:** 10 minutes

This sweet and zesty vinaigrette makes a great salad dressing. It has intense flavor as well as anti-inflammatory ingredients like citrus, herbs, and spices. It can also be used as a marinade for meat or plant-based proteins, like tofu.

Juice of 4 limes
3 tablespoons honey
2 tablespoons apple cider vinegar
2 tablespoons Dijon mustard
2 garlic cloves, minced
3 scallions, finely chopped
½ cup roughly chopped fresh cilantro

In a medium bowl, whisk together the lime juice, honey, vinegar, mustard, and garlic. Add the scallions and cilantro and stir to combine.

✳ **Storage:** Store in a screw-top jar in the refrigerator for up to 5 days.

✳ **Substitution tip:** For a spicier vinaigrette, add ½ teaspoon of chili powder or red pepper flakes.

*Per serving (generous 3 tablespoons): Calories: 82; Total Fat: 1g; Saturated Fat: 0g; Protein: 1g; Total Carbohydrates: 21g; Fiber: 2g; Sugar: 16g; Cholesterol: 0mg*

# Simple Citrus Vinaigrette Dressing

**DAIRY-FREE • GLUTEN-FREE • NIGHTSHADE-FREE • NUT-FREE • SOY-FREE • VEGAN**

**Makes** ½ cup

**Prep time:** 10 minutes

A simple, flavorful dressing balanced with fresh citrus, savory herbs, and apple cider vinegar is perfect for an anti-inflammatory diet plan. Make this dressing ahead and keep it handy in the refrigerator to brighten up greens, grains, or beans.

Juice of 1 lemon

2 tablespoons apple cider vinegar

2 tablespoons olive oil

½ teaspoon Dijon mustard

1 garlic clove, minced

¾ teaspoon salt

1 teaspoon freshly ground black pepper

½ teaspoon dried oregano

½ teaspoon dried thyme

In a medium bowl, whisk together the lemon juice, vinegar, oil, mustard, garlic, salt, pepper, oregano, and thyme.

* **Storage:** Store in a screw-top jar in the refrigerator for up to 10 days.

* **Substitution tip:** Increase or decrease herbs or spices to your preference. Swap in fresh basil, mint, or rosemary if you have access to it—you'll get a slightly stronger flavor and even more antioxidants and vitamins.

*Per serving (generous 1½ tablespoons):* Calories: 54; Total Fat: 5g; Saturated Fat: 1g; Protein: 0g; Total Carbohydrates: 1g; Fiber: 0g; Sugar: 0g; Cholesterol: 0mg

# Fresh Dill Marinade

**DAIRY-FREE • GLUTEN-FREE • NIGHTSHADE-FREE • NUT-FREE • SOY-FREE • VEGETARIAN**
**Makes** 1 cup
**Prep time:** 5 minutes

This versatile, flavor-packed marinade is filled with anti-inflammatory fresh herbs and spices. The garlic and dill combine to create a unique, bold flavor that pairs well with protein-packed main dishes, like salmon or tofu.

⅓ cup olive oil

Juice of ½ lemon

2 tablespoons red wine vinegar

1 tablespoon honey

3 garlic cloves, minced

¼ cup roughly chopped fresh dill

1 teaspoon salt

1 teaspoon freshly ground black pepper

In a medium bowl, whisk together the oil, lemon juice, vinegar, honey, garlic, dill, salt, and pepper.

\* **Storage:** Store in a screw-top jar in the refrigerator for up to 5 days.

\* **Reuse tip:** This marinade is perfect on any seafood. Use it on anti-inflammatory options such as halibut or trout. It also pairs well with other plant-based proteins and mushrooms.

*Per serving (1 tablespoon): Calories: 46; Total Fat: 4g; Saturated Fat: 1g; Protein: 0g; Total Carbohydrates: 2g; Fiber: 0g; Sugar: 1g; Cholesterol: 0mg*

# Zesty Vegan Caesar Dressing

**DAIRY-FREE · GLUTEN-FREE · NIGHTSHADE-FREE · NUT-FREE · SOY-FREE · VEGAN**

**Makes** 1 cup
**Prep time:** 10 minutes

This vegan, anti-inflammatory version of Caesar dressing goes great on salads or wraps. Savory garlic, mustard, and capers combine with rich tahini and are balanced with a touch of maple syrup. Caesar dressing is traditionally garlic-heavy, but feel free to adjust the garlic up or down to taste.

¼ cup tahini

1 teaspoon Dijon mustard

Juice of 1 lemon

2 teaspoons capers, minced

3 garlic cloves, minced

1 teaspoon maple syrup

½ teaspoon salt

½ teaspoon freshly ground black pepper

1 or 2 tablespoons cold water

In a medium bowl, whisk together the tahini, mustard, lemon juice, capers, garlic, maple syrup, salt, and pepper. Add the water 1 tablespoon at a time if needed to thin the dressing to a pourable consistency.

✳ **Storage:** Store in a screw-top jar in the refrigerator for up to 12 days. The dressing will thicken when refrigerated, so to serve, whisk in a little cold water to return it to a pourable consistency.

*Per serving (generous 3 tablespoons): Calories: 82; Total Fat: 7g; Saturated Fat: 1g; Protein: 2g; Total Carbohydrates: 5g; Fiber: 1g; Sugar: 1g; Cholesterol: 0mg*

# Creamy Avocado Dressing

**DAIRY-FREE • GLUTEN-FREE • NIGHTSHADE-FREE • NUT-FREE • SOY-FREE • VEGAN**

**Makes** 1 cup
**Prep time:** 10 minutes

A creamy dressing can absolutely be made vegan—if you use the right ingredients! This avocado-based, anti-inflammatory dressing can be whipped up in a blender or food processor at a moment's notice so you always have a rich, savory dressing for greens.

1 avocado, halved
   and pitted
1 tablespoon olive oil
2 teaspoons apple
   cider vinegar
1 garlic clove, peeled
   but whole
Juice of 1 lemon
½ teaspoon onion
   powder
1 teaspoon maple syrup
1 teaspoon Dijon mustard
½ teaspoon salt
½ teaspoon freshly
   ground black pepper
10 tablespoons
   cold water

Scoop the avocado into a food processor or blender. Add the oil, vinegar, garlic, lemon juice, onion powder, maple syrup, mustard, salt, and pepper and pulse the mixture until it's smooth and creamy. Add as much water as you need, 1 tablespoon at a time, to thin it to a thick but pourable consistency.

✱ **Storage:** Store in a screw-top jar in the refrigerator for up to 5 days.

✱ **Substitution tip:** Want even more flavor? Increase the garlic, salt, and lemon to taste.

***Per serving (generous 3 tablespoons):*** *Calories: 105; Total Fat: 9g; Saturated Fat: 2g; Protein: 1g; Total Carbohydrates: 7g; Fiber: 4g; Sugar: 3g; Cholesterol: 0mg*

# Simple Ginger Teriyaki Sauce

**DAIRY-FREE · GLUTEN-FREE · NUT-FREE · VEGETARIAN**
**Makes** 1 cup
**Prep time:** 5 minutes · **Cook time:** 5 minutes

Store-bought teriyaki sauce can be high in added sugar, artificial colors, and flavors—but not this one! This recipe combines several anti-inflammatory ingredients to create a versatile and flavorful sauce that pairs great with meat, tofu, and vegetables.

¼ cup tamari

3 tablespoons cold water, plus 1½ teaspoons

2 tablespoons honey

2 tablespoons rice vinegar

1 garlic clove, minced

½ teaspoon sriracha

1½ teaspoons grated fresh ginger

1½ teaspoons arrowroot powder or cornstarch

1. In a medium bowl, whisk together the tamari, 3 tablespoons of water, the honey, vinegar, garlic, sriracha, and ginger. Transfer the mixture to a medium saucepan and heat it over medium-high heat.

2. While the tamari mixture is heating, in a small bowl, combine the remaining 1½ teaspoons of water and the arrowroot powder, mixing well to incorporate. Allow the mixture to thicken for at least 2 to 3 minutes.

3. Once the tamari mixture boils, reduce the heat to medium-low and whisk in the arrowroot mixture. Continue to whisk the sauce in the pan for 1 to 2 minutes more, until it thickens slightly. Set it aside. The sauce will thicken further as it cools.

4. There will be some larger pieces of garlic and ginger in this sauce. For a smoother sauce, blend the mixture in a blender for 10 to 20 seconds, until the ginger and garlic are completely incorporated.

\* **Storage:** Store in a screw-top jar in the refrigerator for up to 7 days. To serve, add 1 to 2 teaspoons of water as needed to thin. Microwave for 1 minute or until heated through.

\* **Ingredient tip:** Tamari is a popular gluten-free substitute for soy sauce. Tamari and soy sauce are both high in sodium, but this anti-inflammatory diet plan is low in sodium overall—though there are reduced-sodium versions of soy sauce and tamari available.

*Per serving (generous 3 tablespoons): Calories: 40; Total Fat: 0g; Saturated Fat: 0g; Protein: 2g; Total Carbohydrates: 9g; Fiber: 0g; Sugar: 7g; Cholesterol: 0mg*

# Avocado Crema

**DAIRY-FREE • GLUTEN-FREE • NIGHTSHADE-FREE • NUT-FREE • SOY-FREE • VEGAN**

**Makes** 1 cup
**Prep time:** 5 minutes

This "crema" is vegan-friendly and completely anti-inflammatory. Avocado provides a creamy base that also offers fiber, vitamins, minerals, antioxidants, and heart-healthy monounsaturated fat. Cilantro brightens up this rich topping and lends it a beautiful green hue as well.

1 avocado, halved
   and pitted
¼ cup full-fat
   coconut milk
Juice of 1 lime
¼ teaspoon salt
¼ cup fresh cilantro
   leaves

Scoop the avocado into a food processor or blender. Add the coconut milk, lime juice, salt, and cilantro and pulse the mixture until it's smooth and creamy but still thick in consistency.

✳ **Storage:** Store the crema in a medium storage container in the refrigerator for up to 4 days. To avoid browning, pour a thin layer of olive oil on top of the crema in the container to prevent exposure to air. To serve, pour off the excess olive oil or mix it into the crema.

✳ **Reuse tip:** You will have extra coconut milk in the can after making this recipe. Freeze the rest in ice cube trays and store the cubes in a plastic bag in the freezer, then thaw and toss them into recipes as needed!

***Per serving (¼ cup):*** *Calories: 122; Total Fat: 11g; Saturated Fat: 4g; Protein: 2g; Total Carbohydrates: 7g; Fiber: 4g; Sugar: 2g; Cholesterol: 0mg*

# Homemade Enchilada Sauce

**DAIRY-FREE • NUT-FREE • SOY-FREE • VEGAN**

**Makes** 4½ cups

**Prep time:** 5 minutes • **Cook time:** 15 minutes

Making your own enchilada sauce is quick and easy. This flavorful recipe relies on the vibrant herbs and spices in an anti-inflammatory spice blend to deepen the flavor of a simple tomato sauce. Feel free to adjust proportions here to make the sauce more or less spicy, per your preference.

¼ cup canola oil

¼ cup whole wheat flour

1 (28-ounce) can
   tomato sauce

½ teaspoon maple syrup

⅓ cup Anti-Inflammatory
   Multiuse Spice Blend
   (page 84)

½ cup water, plus
   1 tablespoon, as needed

1. In a medium saucepan, heat the oil over medium-high heat. Whisk in the flour until it's well combined with the oil, about 1 minute.

2. Stir in the tomato sauce, maple syrup, spice blend, and 1 tablespoon of water. Bring the mixture to a boil, then reduce the heat and let simmer until slightly thickened, about 10 minutes.

3. Add water, 1 tablespoon at a time up to ½ cup, as needed to give the sauce a thick but pourable consistency.

✻ **Storage:** Store in a screw-top jar in the refrigerator for up to 5 days. This recipe also freezes well, so you can make a double batch to have for future recipes.

✻ **Substitution tip:** This recipe is tomato-based, so it cannot be made nightshade-free. But you can make it gluten-free by using a gluten-free flour blend instead of whole wheat flour.

*Per serving (generous 1 cup): Calories: 199; Total Fat: 14g; Saturated Fat: 1g; Protein: 3g; Total Carbohydrates: 17g; Fiber: 3g; Sugar: 8g; Cholesterol: 0mg*

# Basic Brown Rice

**DAIRY-FREE • GLUTEN-FREE • NIGHTSHADE-FREE • NUT-FREE • SOY-FREE • VEGAN**

**Makes** 2½ cups

**Prep time:** 10 minutes • **Cook time:** 45 to 55 minutes

Brown rice is an anti-inflammatory meal-prep staple, so you should expect to be using this recipe often! Choose short- or long-grain brown rice, jasmine brown rice, or even wild rice (for the latter, you'll need 1 cup more of water). This simple recipe needs no special equipment. You'll get used to whipping up quick batches in no time.

1 cup brown rice

2½ cups water

½ teaspoon salt

1. In a medium saucepan, combine the rice, water, and salt. Bring the mixture to a simmer, uncovered, over medium-high heat. Reduce the heat to low, cover, and simmer for 45 minutes. Check if the liquid has been absorbed. Do not stir the rice during cooking. If the liquid is not absorbed after 45 minutes, cover it again and continue cooking, checking every 2 minutes to see if the liquid has absorbed. When no liquid remains, remove the pan from the heat and set it aside to cool for 10 minutes.

2. Fluff the rice gently with a fork to avoid sticking.

✴ **Storage:** Store the rice in a storage container in the refrigerator for up to 4 days. Freeze for up to 6 months.

✴ **Cooking tip:** Rice should technically be rinsed before you cook it to remove starch from the surface of the grains, yielding a better cooked texture. You can skip this step to save time, but if you aren't in a rush, rinse your rice in a fine-mesh sieve under cool running water until the water runs clear, usually about 1 minute.

***Per serving (½ cup):*** *Calories: 138; Total Fat: 1g; Saturated Fat: 0g; Protein: 3g; Total Carbohydrates: 29g; Fiber: 1g; Sugar: 0g; Cholesterol: 0mg*

# Savory Herbed Quinoa

**DAIRY-FREE • GLUTEN-FREE • NIGHTSHADE-FREE • NUT-FREE • SOY-FREE • VEGAN**

**Makes** 3½ cups

**Prep time:** 10 minutes • **Cook time:** 20 minutes

Quinoa on its own has a very mild flavor, but prepared with savory herbs and seasoning, it becomes a delicious and versatile side dish. Fresh parsley, basil, and scallions add depth of flavor to this recipe, in addition to anti-inflammatory benefits.

1 cup quinoa, rinsed

2 cups vegetable broth

1½ tablespoons olive oil

Juice of ½ lemon

½ teaspoon salt

½ teaspoon freshly ground black pepper

½ cup chopped fresh parsley

½ cup chopped fresh basil

2 scallions, chopped

1. In a saucepan, combine the quinoa and broth and bring to a boil over high heat. Reduce the heat to medium-low, cover, and simmer for 15 to 20 minutes, or until the liquid is absorbed and the quinoa looks fluffy.
2. Remove from the heat and let rest, covered, for 10 minutes more.
3. Transfer the cooked quinoa to a large bowl and add the olive oil, lemon juice, salt, pepper, parsley, basil, and scallions. Stir to incorporate.

**\* Storage:** Store the quinoa in a storage container in the refrigerator for up to 5 days. Freeze quinoa for up to 2 months and thaw it in the refrigerator overnight before reheating in the microwave.

**\* Reuse tip:** Cook double the amount of quinoa and divide the cooked quinoa in half. Add the herbs in this recipe to one portion and keep the remaining quinoa plain to use in other recipes!

*Per serving (scant ¾ cup): Calories: 175; Total Fat: 6g; Saturated Fat: 1g; Protein: 5g; Total Carbohydrates: 25g; Fiber: 3g; Sugar: 2g; Cholesterol: 0mg*

# Garlic-Herb Marinated Tempeh or Tofu

**DAIRY-FREE • GLUTEN-FREE • NIGHTSHADE-FREE • NUT-FREE • VEGAN**
**Makes** 3 servings
**Prep time:** 10 minutes, plus 20 minutes to marinate • **Cook time:** 20 minutes

Tempeh and tofu have very subtle flavors on their own, but they can be dressed up easily. Marinating these plant-based proteins in savory broth, tangy vinegar, and anti-inflammatory herbs and spices makes a wonderful base for many dishes.

8 ounces tempeh or 14 ounces tofu

2 tablespoons olive oil

¼ cup vegetable broth or water

1 tablespoon white wine vinegar

3 garlic cloves, minced

1½ teaspoons dried thyme

½ teaspoon salt

½ teaspoon freshly ground black pepper

1. Preheat the oven to 400°F. Line a sheet pan with parchment paper.
2. If using tempeh, slice it crosswise into 1-inch-thick slices. If using tofu, press the tops and sides gently with a paper towel to remove extra water. Halve it lengthwise and press the slices again with a paper towel. Cut the tofu into 1-inch cubes.
3. To make the marinade, in a large bowl, combine the oil, broth, vinegar, garlic, thyme, salt, and pepper. Place the tempeh or tofu in the marinade and use a spoon to coat it thoroughly. Let it marinate for at least 10 minutes, then flip or toss and marinate for 10 minutes more.
4. Pour the tofu or tempeh onto the sheet pan in a single layer. Pour any additional marinade onto the pan and bake for 15 to 20 minutes, until the tempeh or tofu is slightly browned.

\* **Storage:** Store in a storage container in the refrigerator for up to 6 days. To serve, microwave for 1 minute.

\* **Reuse tip:** Tempeh and tofu are the perfect proteins for so many recipes. Make a batch—or even a double batch—of this each week and add it to salad or wrap recipes from this book.

*Per serving: Calories: 233; Total Fat: 17g; Saturated Fat: 3g; Protein: 14g; Total Carbohydrates: 9g; Fiber: 0g; Sugar: 0g; Cholesterol: 0mg*

Stovetop Steel-Cut Oats with
Banana, Cherries, and Almonds
*page 101*

CHAPTER

**7**

# Breakfast

# Green Tea Power Smoothie

**DAIRY-FREE • GLUTEN-FREE • NIGHTSHADE-FREE • NUT-FREE • SOY-FREE • VEGAN**

**Makes** 1 serving
**Prep time:** 10 minutes

Green tea is the perfect base for a morning smoothie. It's hydrating and anti-inflammatory due to its dense antioxidant content, and it contains caffeine for an energy boost. Smoothies are a great way to maximize your intake of fruits and veggies, as well as healthy fats and proteins, in the morning. This recipe makes only one serving—for meal-prep purposes, multiply the recipe by 5 (or more) and store the components as smoothie "packs" (see Storage tip) and store in the freezer for later use. Brew the green tea fresh for each smoothie.

1 cup boiling water
1 green tea bag
½ banana, cut up
  and frozen
¼ cup frozen blueberries
1 cup frozen spinach
1 tablespoon chia seeds
3 ice cubes

1. In a large, heatproof measuring cup or bowl, pour the boiling water over the green tea bag. Steep to taste.
2. While the tea steeps, place the frozen banana, blueberries, spinach, and chia seeds in a blender.
3. Drop the ice cubes into the tea to cool it partially. Pour the still-warm tea over the smoothie ingredients and blend until smooth, about 1 minute.

＊ **Storage:** Make smoothie "packs" by storing portions of the banana, berries, greens, and chia seeds together in single-serving freezer bags for up to 2 months. To make a smoothie, simply brew the tea, add ice cubes and the contents of a smoothie pack, and blend.

＊ **Cooking tip:** If using fresh fruit and vegetables for the smoothie packs, freeze them first so they don't stick together in the freezer bags. To do this, freeze the fruits and veggies in a single layer on a baking sheet for 1 to 2 hours. Once frozen, divide into smoothie packs.

＊ **Substitution tip:** Feel free to add nondairy milk such as soy, oat, coconut, or almond, swap in different types of fruit, or add protein powder or silken tofu to boost protein.

*Per serving: Calories: 188; Total Fat: 6g; Saturated Fat: 1g; Protein: 9g; Total Carbohydrates: 31g; Fiber: 12g; Sugar: 12g; Cholesterol: 0mg*

# Fruit and Herb Salad Parfaits

**GLUTEN-FREE · NIGHTSHADE-FREE · SOY-FREE · VEGETARIAN**
**Makes** 3 servings
**Prep time:** 10 minutes

A fruit salad is an anti-inflammatory powerhouse and a satisfying, filling way to start your day. This collection of fruit boosts your fiber, vitamin, and mineral intake first thing in the morning, and it's balanced with anti-inflammatory unsaturated fats and protein. You'll stay full and energized well into your day.

1 cup Ginger-Berry
  Granola (page 72)
1 cup blackberries
1 cup raspberries
1 cup sliced strawberries
1 apple, chopped
2 tangerines or
  clementine
  oranges, segmented
3 large fresh basil
  leaves, chopped
3 large fresh mint
  leaves, chopped
1½ cups plain dairy
  or nondairy yogurt
1 tablespoon honey

1. Prepare the granola as directed.
2. In a large bowl, combine the blackberries, raspberries, strawberries, apple, tangerines, basil, and mint and mix until combined. Portion the fruit salad into 3 screw-top glass jars and top each one with ½ cup of yogurt. Drizzle each with 1 teaspoon of honey and top with ⅓ cup of granola.

\* **Storage:** Store the parfait jars in the refrigerator for up to 2 days. The granola will get soft when it's in contact with the yogurt, so if you want it to stay crunchy, store the granola in a container separate from the yogurt.

\* **Substitution tip:** Make this recipe vegan by substituting agave or maple syrup for honey. Try varying this recipe by adding different toppings, like unsweetened coconut flakes, chia or hemp seeds, or chopped nuts.

*Per serving: Calories: 434; Total Fat: 14g; Saturated Fat: 4g; Protein: 12g; Total Carbohydrates: 70g; Fiber: 13g; Sugar: 40g; Cholesterol: 16mg*

# Cinnamon-Walnut Brown Rice Pudding

**DAIRY-FREE • GLUTEN-FREE • NIGHTSHADE-FREE • SOY-FREE • VEGETARIAN**

**Makes** 4 servings

**Prep time:** 45 minutes • **Cook time:** 20 minutes

This warming, comforting rice pudding is a healthy twist on a classic. Low in added sugar and high in antioxidants and complex carbohydrates, this brown rice dish will fuel your morning. Cinnamon and omega-3-rich walnuts give this recipe depth of flavor and texture. Use soy milk for higher protein content.

Basic Brown Rice
   (page 93)
2 cups unsweetened
   nondairy milk, divided
⅓ cup maple syrup
¼ teaspoon salt
1 large egg, beaten
½ teaspoon pure
   vanilla extract
½ teaspoon ground
   cinnamon
¼ cup chopped walnuts

1. Prepare the brown rice as directed.
2. In a saucepan, combine the rice with 1½ cups of milk, the maple syrup, and salt. Cook over medium heat for 15 to 20 minutes, or until thick.
3. Pour in the remaining ½ cup of milk and the egg. Continue cooking for 2 to 3 minutes, stirring constantly. Remove the pudding from the heat and stir in the vanilla, cinnamon, and walnuts.
4. Portion the rice pudding into 4 medium storage containers.

**\*** **Storage:** Store in the refrigerator for up to 4 days. To serve, microwave for 1 to 2 minutes until heated through. Garnish with a sprinkle of cinnamon or chopped walnuts, if desired.

**\*** **Reuse tip:** You can store extra brown rice in the freezer for convenient use in recipes like this one. For this recipe, feel free to use the rice straight from the freezer—no need to thaw it first.

***Per serving:*** *Calories: 339; Total Fat: 9g; Saturated Fat: 1g; Protein: 10g; Total Carbohydrates: 54g; Fiber: 2g; Sugar: 21g; Cholesterol: 47mg*

# Stovetop Steel-Cut Oats with Banana, Cherries, and Almonds

**DAIRY-FREE • GLUTEN-FREE • NIGHTSHADE-FREE • SOY-FREE • VEGAN**

**Makes** 5 servings

**Prep time:** 5 minutes • **Cook time:** 15 minutes

You can whip up hearty oats on the stove in less than 30 minutes. Naturally sweetened with banana, these steel-cut oats are full of fiber and are complemented by delicious anti-inflammatory cherries and almonds. To save time, cook the oats ahead, and you can have this recipe done in barely 5 minutes!

2 cups steel-cut oats

4½ cups nondairy milk

1 very ripe large banana, fresh or frozen

2 cups cherries, fresh or frozen, halved and pitted

½ cup slivered almonds, chopped

1. In a saucepan, combine the oats and milk and bring to a boil over medium-high heat. Reduce the heat to medium-low and simmer for 15 minutes, or until the oats are soft.
2. Remove from the heat and add the banana. Cover the pot so that the banana softens in the trapped heat. Mash or stir the softened banana into the oats until incorporated. Add the cherries and almonds, mixing to combine.
3. Cool the oats completely, then portion it into 5 screw-top glass jars and garnish with more cherries or almonds, if desired.

\* **Storage:** Store in the refrigerator for up to 4 days. To serve, add 1 to 2 tablespoons of milk to the oats to thin the mixture slightly and microwave it for 1 to 2 minutes until heated through.

\* **Substitution tip:** Swap in rolled oats instead of steel-cut oats for a softer, more traditional oatmeal texture. To do this, reduce the cooking time to 10 minutes. For a sweeter flavor, add an extra ½ banana.

*Per serving: Calories: 380; Total Fat: 11g; Saturated Fat: 1g; Protein: 14g; Total Carbohydrates: 55g; Fiber: 9g; Sugar: 20g; Cholesterol: 0mg*

# Simple No-Grain Banana Pancakes with Fruit Compote

**DAIRY-FREE • GLUTEN-FREE • NIGHTSHADE-FREE • NUT-FREE • SOY-FREE • VEGETARIAN**
**Makes** 2 servings
**Prep time:** 10 minutes • **Cook time:** 5 minutes

Did you know that pancakes can be healthy? These no-grain banana pancakes are naturally gluten- and grain-free and high in protein. There's no maple syrup served with these pancakes; instead, you'll use anti-inflammatory and naturally sweet fruit compote.

2 cups berries
    (strawberries,
    blueberries, or
    cherries), fresh
    or frozen
Juice of 1 medium orange
2 bananas, mashed
2 large eggs, beaten
¼ teaspoon baking soda
1 tablespoon coconut oil

1. In a small saucepan, combine the berries and orange juice. Bring to a boil over medium-high heat. Reduce the heat to medium-low and cook for 10 to 12 minutes, stirring occasionally with a whisk or masher and mashing the fruit, until the mixture thickens slightly. Remove from the heat. The mixture will thicken more as it cools.

2. While the compote cooks, in a medium bowl, combine the bananas, eggs, and baking soda, mixing with a wooden spoon to incorporate.

3. In a large skillet, heat the coconut oil over medium-high heat until hot. Pour the pancake batter into the pan, using ¼ cup of batter for each pancake. Cook the pancakes until they puff up slightly, appear set in the middle, and the edges become translucent, 4 to 5 minutes. Gently flip the pancakes and cook for 1 to 2 minutes more.

4. Portion the cooled pancakes into 2 storage containers. Transfer the compote to a screw-top glass jar.

✳ **Storage:** Store pancakes in the refrigerator for 1 to 2 days. Store the compote for up to 5 days. To serve, microwave the pancakes in 30-second intervals until heated through. Microwave the compote for 30 seconds and pour it on top of the pancakes.

*Per serving: Calories: 321; Total Fat: 13g; Saturated Fat: 8g; Protein: 9g; Total Carbohydrates: 48g; Fiber: 8g; Sugar: 29g; Cholesterol: 186mg*

# Tofu Scramble with Veggies

**DAIRY-FREE · GLUTEN-FREE · NIGHTSHADE-FREE · NUT-FREE · VEGAN**
**Makes** 2 servings
**Prep time:** 5 minutes · **Cook time:** 10 minutes

Tofu scrambles as well as eggs do, so start your day with a protein-packed scramble full of your favorite flavorful vegetables. Flavored with turmeric, a potent anti-inflammatory herb, this scramble will take on a vibrant yellow color and rich flavor. Feel free to swap in whichever antioxidant-dense vegetables you enjoy the most.

1 tablespoon olive oil
½ medium yellow
    onion, diced
1 garlic clove, minced
1 cup chopped asparagus
1 cup baby spinach,
    chopped
1 (8-ounce) block
    firm tofu, pressed
    with paper towels
    and crumbled
½ teaspoon ground
    turmeric
½ teaspoon salt
½ teaspoon freshly
    ground black pepper

1. In a large skillet, heat the oil over medium heat. Add the onion, garlic, and asparagus and sauté for 3 to 5 minutes, until the onions are translucent and the asparagus has softened. Add the baby spinach and cook, stirring constantly, until it reduces in size and incorporates into the mixture.
2. Add the tofu and continue to sauté over medium heat for 4 to 5 minutes, until the tofu browns slightly. If the tofu sticks to the pan, add a small splash of water and use a spatula to scrape up the stuck bits. Add the turmeric, salt, and pepper and stir to combine. Remove from the heat.
3. Portion the scramble into 2 storage containers.

\* **Storage:** Store the tofu scramble in the refrigerator for up to 5 days. To serve, microwave for 1 to 2 minutes until heated through.

\* **Substitution tip:** Mix up this scramble by using other veggies. Try peppers, tomatoes, scallions, avocado, broccoli, zucchini, sweet potato, or squash. You can also add some shredded cheese or a vegan cheese alternative. Garnish with nutritional yeast, salsa, or hot sauce for additional flavor.

*Per serving:* Calories: 258; Total Fat: 17g; Saturated Fat: 2g; Protein: 20g; Total Carbohydrates: 12g; Fiber: 5g; Sugar: 3g; Cholesterol: 0mg

# Zucchini Breakfast Muffins

**DAIRY-FREE · NIGHTSHADE-FREE · NUT-FREE · SOY-FREE · VEGETARIAN**
**Makes** 12 muffins
**Prep time:** 10 minutes · **Cook time:** 20 minutes

Zucchini is the secret ingredient in these breakfast muffins, boosting your mornings with fiber, vitamins, minerals, and antioxidants. There's no need to start your day with sugar-filled pastries when a whole-grain, naturally sweetened, secretly veggie-packed option is so easy to whip up. Feel free to swap in a gluten-free all-purpose flour to make these gluten-free.

2 cups grated zucchini
  (about 2 small zucchini)
1 cup whole wheat flour
1 cup all-purpose flour
1 teaspoon
  baking powder
1 teaspoon baking soda
1 teaspoon ground
  cinnamon
½ teaspoon salt
2 large eggs
½ cup maple syrup
½ cup unsweetened
  nondairy milk (oat,
  almond, or soy)
¼ cup grapeseed
  or avocado oil
1 teaspoon pure
  vanilla extract

1. Preheat the oven to 375°F. Line a 12-cup muffin tin with paper or silicone liners.
2. Press the grated zucchini gently between paper towels to remove excess moisture. Set it aside.
3. In a large bowl, whisk together the whole wheat flour, all-purpose flour, baking powder, baking soda, cinnamon, and salt.
4. In a medium bowl, whisk together the eggs, maple syrup, milk, oil, and vanilla. Pour the egg mixture into the flour mixture and stir with a wooden spoon to combine. Gently fold in the zucchini, until just incorporated.
5. Divide the batter evenly among the muffin cups and bake for 18 to 20 minutes, or until the muffin tops are firm to the touch.
6. Let the muffins cool, then transfer them to a large storage container.

✳ **Storage:** Refrigerate the muffins for up to 3 days, or freeze them for up to 3 months. To serve, microwave for 30 seconds to 1 minute.

✳ **Substitution tip:** Add mix-ins to taste. When adding the zucchini, blend in ½ cup of chopped walnuts, raisins, or dried cranberries.

*Per serving (2 muffins): Calories: 338; Total Fat: 12g; Saturated Fat: 2g; Protein: 8g; Total Carbohydrates: 52g; Fiber: 4g; Sugar: 18g; Cholesterol: 62mg*

# Chile-Cumin Scrambled Eggs

**DAIRY-FREE • GLUTEN-FREE • NUT-FREE • SOY-FREE • VEGETARIAN**
**Makes** 2 servings
**Prep time:** 10 minutes • **Cook time:** 10 minutes

Scrambled eggs make a lovely vehicle for veggies and anti-inflammatory spices. Brighten up your average scramble by adding savory cumin and vibrant chiles before serving. Enjoy this scramble on toast, wrapped in a tortilla, with a side of fruit, or, best of all, with Roasted Red Potatoes with Herbs (page 154).

½ recipe Roasted Red
  Potatoes with Herbs
2 teaspoons olive oil
¼ medium yellow
  onion, diced
1 garlic clove, minced
¼ teaspoon salt
¼ teaspoon freshly
  ground black pepper
¼ teaspoon
  ground cumin
⅛ teaspoon chili powder
4 large eggs, beaten
1 (4-ounce) can diced
  mild green chiles,
  drained of excess juice

1. Prepare the red potatoes as directed and put them in the oven.
2. In a large skillet, heat the oil over medium heat. Add the onion and garlic and sauté for 3 to 4 minutes, until the onion is translucent.
3. Add the salt, pepper, cumin, and chili powder, mixing them into the onion mixture for about 30 seconds. Add the eggs and chiles. Use a wooden spoon to scramble the mixture quickly and constantly so that the eggs cook evenly. Continue cooking for 3 to 5 minutes, until the eggs are no longer wet but before they begin to brown. Remove from the heat.
4. Remove the potatoes from the oven and cool before storing.
5. Portion the potatoes and eggs separately in 2 storage containers each.

✳ **Storage:** Store in the refrigerator for up to 3 days. To serve, microwave the scramble until warm in 10-second intervals to avoid making them tough. Microwave the potatoes for 1 to 2 minutes.

✳ **Cooking tip:** If you do some of the prep work ahead, you can always make a quick fresh scramble. Prep the onion and garlic and put together the spices and store them in portions to use later in the week. When ready to serve, cook a portion of the onion and garlic as directed (step 2) and scramble in 2 fresh eggs and the chiles.

***Per serving:*** *Calories: 391; Total Fat: 21g; Saturated Fat: 5g; Protein: 15g; Total Carbohydrates: 34g; Fiber: 5g; Sugar: 5g; Cholesterol: 372mg*

# Fiesta Breakfast Bowls with Black Beans and Savory Herbed Quinoa

**DAIRY-FREE • GLUTEN-FREE • NIGHTSHADE-FREE • NUT-FREE • SOY-FREE • VEGETARIAN**
**Makes** 3 servings
**Prep time:** 15 minutes • **Cook time:** 15 minutes

A breakfast bowl is a quick, healthy, and easy on-the-go breakfast to take to work or school. This fiesta bowl boasts bright colors and bold flavors from anti-inflammatory vegetables and savory spices, plus fiber and protein from black beans, quinoa, and hard-boiled eggs. If you're not nightshade-free, add salsa or hot sauce as a garnish.

1 cup Savory Herbed
  Quinoa (page 94)
3 large eggs
1 (15.5-ounce) can
  black beans, drained
  and rinsed
½ teaspoon
  ground cumin
Juice of 1 lime
1½ cups baby spinach
Salt
Freshly ground
  black pepper
1 small avocado, sliced
¼ cup chopped
  fresh cilantro

1. Prepare the quinoa as directed.
2. Place the eggs in a medium pot and cover with water so that they're completely submerged. Bring the water to a boil over high heat. When the water boils, remove the pot from the heat, cover, and let sit for 11 minutes. Drain the water and set the eggs aside to cool.
3. While the eggs are cooking, in a large saucepan, combine the black beans, cumin, and lime juice and stir over medium heat until the mixture is heated through, 3 to 5 minutes. Remove from the heat and let cool.
4. If serving right away, line the bottom of each bowl with ½ cup of spinach, then top one half of each bowl with quinoa and the other half with black beans. Peel and halve the eggs and place two halves on top of each bowl. Add salt and pepper to taste. Garnish with avocado and cilantro.
5. If storing for later, store the quinoa and beans together in 3 medium storage containers. Store the spinach in a separate large container and the cilantro and avocado together in 3 separate small containers or baggies. Store the eggs in their shells.

\* **Storage:** Refrigerate all the components for up to 5 days. To serve, follow the assembly instructions in step 4.

*Per serving: Calories: 267; Total Fat: 13g; Saturated Fat: 3g; Protein: 14g; Total Carbohydrates: 4g; Fiber: 10g; Sugar: 2g; Cholesterol: 140mg*

# Simple Breakfast Wraps

**GLUTEN-FREE • NIGHTSHADE-FREE • NUT-FREE • VEGETARIAN**
**Makes** 4 wraps
**Prep time:** 10 minutes • **Cook time:** 5 minutes

Not all breakfasts are good to make ahead, but these simple and savory, meal prep-friendly breakfast wraps certainly are. This adaptable recipe uses eggs or tofu as its base. Add in any of your own favorite spices and herbs. This recipe uses cheese, but you can easily eliminate it or use nutritional yeast instead.

1 teaspoon olive oil
4 large eggs or
   1 (14-ounce) block
   firm tofu
½ teaspoon salt
½ teaspoon freshly
   ground black pepper
2 cups baby spinach
4 tablespoons crumbled
   feta cheese
4 (8-inch) tortillas,
   gluten-free or
   whole wheat

1. In a large skillet, warm the oil over medium heat. Add the eggs or tofu, salt, pepper, and spinach. Scramble the mixture, stirring constantly (and breaking up the tofu, if using), for 3 to 5 minutes, until the eggs are cooked (or the tofu is warmed through) and the spinach has reduced in size and incorporated into the mixture.
2. To assemble the wraps, spread 1 tablespoon of feta in the middle of each tortilla. Divide the egg or tofu and spinach mixture among the tortillas on top of the feta, then wrap the tortillas as you would a burrito, folding the sides in, folding the bottom, and then tucking the top down. Let the wraps cool.
3. Roll each wrap in foil.

＊ **Storage:** Store in the refrigerator for up to 4 days. To freeze, wrap in foil and store for up to 2 months. To serve, remove foil and microwave for 1 to 2 minutes. Thaw frozen wraps in the refrigerator overnight before reheating.

＊ **Substitution tip:** Make this recipe your own by adding different vegetables and cheese. Feel free to swap in peppers, tomatoes, broccoli, zucchini, asparagus, mushrooms, or onions, or use another type of greens, such as kale.

***Per serving (1 wrap):*** *Calories: 238; Total Fat: 12g; Saturated Fat: 5g; Protein: 12g; Total Carbohydrates: 20g; Fiber: 5g; Sugar: 2g; Cholesterol: 194mg*

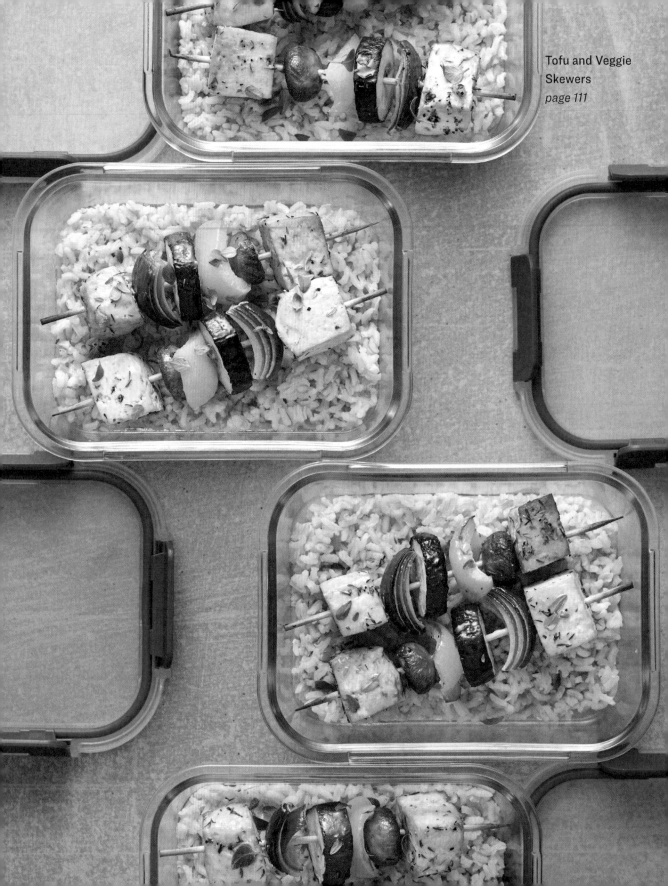

Tofu and Veggie
Skewers
*page 111*

# Lunch

# Protein Lunch Smoothie Packs with Berries and Greens

**DAIRY-FREE • GLUTEN-FREE • NIGHTSHADE-FREE • VEGAN**
**Makes** 4 smoothies
**Prep time:** 5 minutes

Smoothies aren't just for breakfast—they make a great quick lunch to keep your energy up and your blood sugar levels stable. This delicious, filling, all-natural smoothie combines whole-food protein from silken tofu, filling complex carbs from oats, and inflammation-calming antioxidants from fruits and veggies. Freeze the ingredients in smoothie "packs," add milk and tofu, and blend them up in seconds!

1 cup old-fashioned rolled oats

2 bananas, halved and frozen

1⅓ cups frozen strawberries

2 cups spinach

6 cups unsweetened almond or oat milk

16 ounces silken tofu

1. To each of 4 freezer bags, add ¼ cup of oats, half a banana, ⅓ cup of strawberries, and ½ cup of spinach. Store the smoothie packs in the freezer.
2. To make a single smoothie, in a blender, combine 1½ cups of milk and 4 ounces of tofu. Add the contents of 1 smoothie pack and blend until smooth and creamy.

✱ **Storage:** Freeze smoothie packs for up to 4 months. You can refrigerate a prepared smoothie in a screw-top glass jar for up to 3 days and reblend before serving, adding 1 to 2 tablespoons of milk to thin it if necessary.

✱ **Substitution tip:** If you're soy-free, replace the tofu in this recipe with a plant-based protein powder or nut butter, like peanut or almond butter.

*Per Serving (1 smoothie): Calories: 475; Total Fat: 11g; Saturated Fat: 1g; Protein: 19g; Total Carbohydrates: 81g; Fiber: 10g; Sugar: 29g; Cholesterol: 0mg*

# Tofu and Veggie Skewers

**DAIRY-FREE • GLUTEN-FREE • NIGHTSHADE-FREE • NUT-FREE • VEGAN**

**Makes** 8 skewers (4 servings)
**Prep time:** 20 minutes • **Cook time:** 30 minutes

In this recipe, tofu and veggies are marinated in a homemade, all-natural sauce and then oven-baked on skewers in a delicious, hands-free preparation style that's ultra-portable and fun to eat. Serve over brown rice for a balanced, filling meal.

Garlic-Herb Marinated
  Tempeh or Tofu
  (page 95)
Basic Brown Rice
  (page 93)
½ red onion, cut into
  large chunks
1 medium zucchini, cut
  into ½-inch-thick slices
1 yellow squash or yellow
  bell pepper, cut into
  ½-inch-thick slices
1 (8-ounce) package
  mushrooms,
  stems removed

1. Marinate the tofu for 20 minutes as directed.
2. Soak 8 (6-inch) wooden skewers in water (so they don't char in the oven) for 20 minutes.
3. Meanwhile, start the brown rice as directed.
4. Preheat the oven to 425°F. Line a large sheet pan with parchment paper.
5. To make the skewers, slide marinated tofu slices (reserve the marinade), chunks of onion, zucchini slices, squash slices, and mushrooms in an alternating pattern onto the skewers, leaving 1 inch of skewer empty on each end.
6. Transfer the skewers to the pan and drizzle half of the reserved tofu marinade over them. Set the remaining marinade aside. Bake the skewers for 20 minutes, then flip them and coat with the remaining marinade. Bake for 15 to 20 minutes more, until the tofu has browned and the vegetables are soft.
7. Remove the brown rice from the heat and set it aside to cool.
8. Portion the cooled brown rice into 4 large containers and place 2 skewers in each.

\* **Storage:** Store in the refrigerator for up to 5 days. To reheat, microwave for 1 to 2 minutes. Roasted vegetables don't freeze well, so this dish is best if consumed within the week.

\* **Substitution tip:** Swap in any vegetable you prefer, such as bell peppers, cherry tomatoes, eggplant, or carrots. You can also use tempeh in place of tofu.

*Per Serving (2 skewers): Calories: 417; Total Fat: 18g; Saturated Fat: 3g; Protein: 20g; Total Carbohydrates: 45g; Fiber: 3g; Sugar: 4g; Cholesterol: 0mg*

# Ginger-Turmeric Carrot Soup

**DAIRY-FREE • GLUTEN-FREE • NIGHTSHADE-FREE • NUT-FREE • SOY-FREE • VEGAN**

**Makes** 5 servings
**Prep time:** 10 minutes • **Cook time:** 40 minutes

This pureed soup is full of anti-inflammatory nutrients that add depth of flavor. Carrots create an earthy, creamy base and pair well with sweet butternut squash. Packaged precut butternut squash (usually found in the refrigerated or freezer section of grocery stores) will save you a lot of time and effort in this recipe. Pair this soup with any of the salads in this book.

2 tablespoons olive oil

4 medium carrots, chopped

1 cup cubed butternut squash

½ yellow onion, diced

2 garlic cloves, minced

1-inch piece fresh ginger, grated

1 tablespoon ground turmeric

1 teaspoon salt

1 teaspoon freshly ground black pepper

3 cups vegetable broth

1 (13.5-ounce) can lite coconut milk

⅓ cup chopped fresh parsley leaves

1. In a large pot, heat the oil over medium heat. Add the carrots, squash, and onion and stir occasionally for 5 to 7 minutes, until the vegetables start to soften and the onions become translucent.
2. Add the garlic, ginger, turmeric, salt, and pepper and stir constantly to combine for 2 minutes more. Add the broth and coconut milk, then bring the mixture to a boil. Reduce the heat to medium-low, cover the pot, and simmer the soup for 20 minutes.
3. Once the vegetables are soft, puree the soup in batches in a stand blender (or in the pot with an immersion blender) until smooth. Allow to cool before storing.
4. Portion the soup into 5 medium storage containers. Store the parsley in a separate container.

✳ **Storage:** Store the soup in the refrigerator for up to 5 days, or freeze it for up to 3 months. To serve, microwave for 2 minutes, stirring well after 1 minute, until heated through. Garnish with parsley.

✳ **Substitution tip:** I use lite coconut milk in this recipe, but feel free to swap in full-fat milk for extra creaminess or calories. Or use soy milk or oat milk instead.

*Per Serving: Calories: 277; Total Fat: 24g; Saturated Fat: 17g; Protein: 3g; Total Carbohydrates: 17g; Fiber: 4g; Sugar: 7g; Cholesterol: 0mg*

# Vegan Sweet Potato and Corn Chowder

**DAIRY-FREE · GLUTEN-FREE · NIGHTSHADE-FREE · NUT-FREE · VEGAN**
**Makes** 5 servings
**Prep time:** 10 minutes · **Cook time:** 40 minutes

Regular chowder is heavy in saturated fat from butter and cream. Luckily, there's another way to make a chowder that's anti-inflammatory and still savory, rich, and delicious. Sweet potato, corn, and protein-packed soy milk create a rich, creamy base for this naturally vegan dish.

3 tablespoons olive oil

1 large yellow onion, diced

1 large leek, both white and green parts, sliced into thin rounds

3 large sweet potatoes, peeled and diced

1 tablespoon water

½ teaspoon dried thyme

1 teaspoon salt

1 teaspoon freshly ground black pepper

4 cups vegetable broth

1 cup unsweetened soy milk

4 cups corn kernels, fresh, canned, or frozen

8 fresh basil leaves, chopped

1. In a large pot, heat the oil over medium heat. Add the onion, leek, and sweet potatoes and cook, stirring occasionally, for 6 to 8 minutes, or until the vegetables start to soften and the onions become translucent. If the mixture is sticking to the pan, add water 1 teaspoon at a time and scrape up the stuck bits with a wooden spoon.

2. Add the thyme, salt, and pepper and cook for 2 minutes more, stirring constantly to combine. Add the broth, increase the heat to high, and bring the mixture to a boil. Reduce the heat to medium-low, cover, and simmer for 30 to 35 minutes, or until the sweet potatoes are tender.

3. Stir in the soy milk. Puree the soup in batches in a stand blender (or in the pot with an immersion blender) until smooth. Return the puree to the pot and add the corn. If the corn is frozen, stir it over medium heat for 5 to 10 minutes to thaw. Cool before storing.

4. Portion the soup into 5 medium storage containers. Store the basil in a separate small container.

✳ **Storage:** Store the soup in the refrigerator for up to 5 days, or freeze it for up to 3 months. To reheat, microwave for 2 minutes, stirring well after 1 minute, until heated through. Garnish with basil.

✳ **Ingredient tip:** If you are soy-free, use oat milk instead. Soy and oat milks contain a higher amount of protein than coconut, almond, or rice milks.

*Per Serving: Calories: 331; Total Fat: 11g; Saturated Fat: 2g; Protein: 8g; Total Carbohydrates: 57g; Fiber: 7g; Sugar: 9g; Cholesterol: 6mg*

# Savory White Bean Soup

**DAIRY-FREE • GLUTEN-FREE • NIGHTSHADE-FREE • NUT-FREE • VEGAN**
**Makes** 5 servings
**Prep time:** 5 minutes • **Cook time:** 20 minutes

Bean soup is the perfect way to maximize protein and fiber as well as anti-inflammatory vitamins, minerals, and antioxidants. Savory garlic and rosemary create earthy undertones that make this delicious and filling soup perfect for any time of year. Bean soup freezes well, so make a batch (or even double it!) and freeze it to grab for lunch whenever you need it.

2 tablespoons olive oil

1 large yellow onion, diced

3 garlic cloves, minced

½ teaspoon dried rosemary

½ teaspoon dried thyme

1 teaspoon salt

¾ teaspoon freshly ground black pepper

1 tablespoon water

4 cups vegetable broth

3 (15.5-ounce) cans white beans (great northern or cannellini), drained and rinsed

½ cup chopped fresh parsley leaves

1. In a large pot, heat the oil over medium heat. Add the onion and cook for 4 to 6 minutes, stirring occasionally, until the onions become translucent and soft. Add the garlic and sauté for 2 minutes more, or until the garlic is soft and fragrant.
2. Add the rosemary, thyme, salt, and pepper and cook for 2 minutes more, stirring constantly to combine. If the mixture is sticking to the pan, add water 1 teaspoon at a time and scrape up the stuck bits with a wooden spoon. Add the broth and beans. Increase the heat to high and bring the mixture to a boil. Then, reduce the heat to medium-low, cover, and simmer for 20 minutes.
3. Using an immersion blender or a potato masher, blend or mash about half of the soup, leaving the other half with texture. Cool before storing.
4. Portion the soup into 5 medium storage containers. Store the parsley in a separate small container.

✳ **Storage:** Store the soup in the refrigerator for up to 5 days, or freeze it for up to 3 months. To serve, microwave for 2 minutes, stirring well after 1 minute, until heated through. Garnish with parsley.

✳ **Ingredient tip:** When purchasing vegetable broth, read the ingredients to ensure it doesn't contain nightshades like tomato if you're avoiding that category of foods.

*Per Serving: Calories: 263; Total Fat: 6g; Saturated Fat: 1g; Protein: 14g; Total Carbohydrates: 39g; Fiber: 12g; Sugar: 3g; Cholesterol: 0mg*

# Bean, Corn, and Quinoa Salad

**DAIRY-FREE • GLUTEN-FREE • NIGHTSHADE-FREE • NUT-FREE • SOY-FREE • VEGAN**
**Makes** 5 servings
**Prep time:** 5 minutes • **Cook time:** 20 minutes

This highly adaptable salad is the perfect make-ahead dish to fill you up all week. It's full of protein and fiber from beans, corn, and whole-grain quinoa. Add different veggies and play around with the seasonings for never-ending variety. A simple dressing makes flavors in this dish pop while anti-inflammatory herbs add health benefits and a light, refreshing taste.

1 cup quinoa, rinsed

2 cups water

½ cup diced red onion

2½ tablespoons olive oil

Juice of 2 limes

2 teaspoons
   ground cumin

1 teaspoon salt

1 teaspoon freshly ground
   black pepper

1½ cups corn kernels,
   fresh or frozen

2 (15.5-ounce) cans
   black beans, drained
   and rinsed

½ cup chopped
   fresh cilantro

3 avocados, halved

1. In a saucepan, combine the quinoa and water and bring it to a boil over high heat. Reduce the heat to medium-low, cover, and cook for 15 minutes, or until the water is absorbed and the quinoa is fluffy.
2. Meanwhile, in a large bowl, combine the onion, oil, lime juice, cumin, salt, and pepper.
3. Transfer the cooked quinoa to the bowl and add the corn and beans. Mix well to coat evenly and cool before storing.
4. Portion the quinoa salad into 5 medium storage containers. Portion the cilantro and half an avocado into each of 5 small containers. (Save the remaining half avocado for another recipe or for another use.)

**✱ Storage:** Store the salad in the refrigerator for up to 5 days. Serve it cold or microwave for 1 to 2 minutes and garnish with the cilantro and avocado.

***Per Serving:*** *Calories: 498; Total Fat: 20g; Saturated Fat: 3g; Protein: 18g; Total Carbohydrates: 69g; Fiber: 19g; Sugar: 4g; Cholesterol: 0mg*

# Lemony Lentil Salad

**DAIRY-FREE • GLUTEN-FREE • NIGHTSHADE-FREE • NUT-FREE • SOY-FREE • VEGAN**
**Makes** 5 servings
**Prep time:** 10 minutes • **Cook time:** 40 minutes

Lentils are the perfect anti-inflammatory addition to a salad. This simple lentil dish is brightened up with fragrant citrus vinaigrette. To ensure that the salad keeps well all week long, I've opted for sturdier lentils, such as black, brown, and French green lentils. Other lentils (especially red) will cook more quickly, but will have a softer texture.

2 cups black, brown, or French green lentils, rinsed
4 cups vegetable broth
Simple Citrus Vinaigrette Dressing (page 86)
10 cups salad greens of your choice
¼ cup chopped fresh dill

1. In a large pot, combine the lentils and broth and bring to a boil over high heat. Reduce the heat to medium-low and simmer for 25 to 30 minutes, until the lentils are soft and the water is absorbed.
2. Meanwhile, make the vinaigrette as directed.
3. When the lentils are finished, pour the dressing over the lentils in the pot and stir well to coat. Let cool.
4. Portion the dressed lentils into 5 medium storage containers. Portion 2 cups of salad greens into each of 5 separate medium containers. Store the dill in 5 separate small containers.

\* **Storage:** Refrigerate all components for up to 5 days. Reheat the lentil salad for 1 to 2 minutes and serve on top of salad greens. Garnish with fresh dill. Cooked lentils can be frozen for up to 3 months; to thaw, let them sit in the refrigerator overnight.

\* **Reuse tip:** This recipe also tastes delicious over Basic Brown Rice (page 93) or Savory Herbed Quinoa (page 94).

*Per Serving: Calories: 420; Total Fat: 7g; Saturated Fat: 1g; Protein: 23g; Total Carbohydrates: 68g; Fiber: 18g; Sugar: 5g; Cholesterol: 0mg*

# Creamy Bean Pasta Salad with Fresh Vegetables

**DAIRY-FREE • GLUTEN-FREE • NIGHTSHADE-FREE • NUT-FREE • SOY-FREE • VEGAN**

**Makes** 4 servings

**Prep time:** 10 minutes • **Cook time:** 12 minutes

If you haven't tried bean pasta yet, now's the time! It's higher in fiber and protein than whole wheat pasta but has nearly the same flavor and texture—plus, it's naturally gluten-free. If you're not avoiding gluten, feel free to swap in whole wheat pasta. The creamy, vegan dressing in this pasta salad complements all the fresh, fiber-rich, anti-inflammatory vegetables in the dish.

1 (8-ounce) package bean pasta (such as chickpea), rotini or elbow shapes

Creamy Avocado Dressing (page 89)

1 (15.5-ounce) can chickpeas, drained and rinsed

12 kalamata olives, pitted and chopped

¼ cup diced red onion

1 medium cucumber, diced

1 large celery stalk, diced

¼ cup chopped fresh parsley

1. Bring a large pot of water to a boil over high heat. Cook the pasta according to package instructions, erring toward al dente (usually 8 to 10 minutes). Drain and let cool.
2. Meanwhile, make the avocado dressing as directed.
3. In a large bowl, combine the chickpeas, olives, onion, cucumber, celery, and avocado dressing and stir with a wooden spoon to thoroughly coat. Add the pasta and gently stir until it's just combined with the other ingredients. Add the parsley and stir until just incorporated.
4. Portion into 4 medium storage containers.

**✳ Storage:** Cooked pasta refrigerates well. Store in the refrigerator for up to 5 days. Serve cold for an on-the-go lunch, dinner, or snack.

**✳ Substitution tip:** You can swap out the red onion for scallions for a subtler flavor. If you're not avoiding nightshades, add cherry tomatoes or diced bell pepper. Or swap out the avocado dressing for the Zesty Vegan Caesar Dressing (page 88).

***Per Serving:*** *Calories: 419; Total Fat: 14g; Saturated Fat: 3g; Protein: 10g; Total Carbohydrates: 67g; Fiber: 15g; Sugar: 7g; Cholesterol: 0mg*

# Quinoa and Apple Protein Bowls

**DAIRY-FREE • GLUTEN-FREE • NIGHTSHADE-FREE • NUT-FREE • VEGAN**

**Makes** 4 servings

**Prep time:** 5 minutes • **Cook time:** 15 minutes

This salad combines protein-packed tofu and whole-grain quinoa with plenty of fresh greens and sweet apples to add even more vitamins, minerals, and antioxidants. Quinoa freezes well, so feel free to prep and freeze quinoa ahead of time to save yourself some time making this dish.

1 (14-ounce) block firm or extra-firm tofu

1 cup quinoa, rinsed

2 cups water

⅓ cup olive oil

¼ cup apple cider vinegar

2 teaspoons Dijon mustard

1 teaspoon maple syrup

½ teaspoon salt

½ teaspoon freshly ground black pepper

3 cups baby spinach or chopped romaine lettuce

1 medium apple, chopped

1. Drain the liquid from the tofu. Press the tofu gently on all sides with paper towels or a clean kitchen towel. Cut it in half horizontally. Slice it into 6 thick strips, then cut those crosswise in the opposite direction, 4 times, to make cubes.

2. In a pot, combine the quinoa and water and bring to a boil over high heat. Reduce the heat to medium-low, cover, and cook for 15 minutes, or until the water is absorbed and the quinoa is fluffy. Remove from the heat and let cool.

3. Meanwhile, in a medium bowl, whisk together the oil, vinegar, mustard, maple syrup, salt, and pepper.

4. If serving right away, fill each of 4 bowls with ¾ cup of greens and top with one portion of the quinoa. Top the quinoa with one-quarter of the chopped apple and one-quarter of the cubed tofu. Drizzle with dressing.

5. If storing for later, portion the quinoa, apple, tofu, and greens into 4 medium containers. Divide the dressing equally into 4 separate small containers.

✳ **Storage:** Refrigerate all components for up to 5 days. To serve, follow assembly instructions in step 4.

✳ **Substitution tip:** If you want to use a grain other than quinoa, you can substitute Basic Brown Rice (page 93). If you want a protein other than tofu, try sliced tempeh for a firmer texture. If you want to forgo soy, use chickpeas instead.

*Per Serving: Calories: 444; Total Fat: 26g; Saturated Fat: 3g; Protein: 17g; Total Carbohydrates: 39g; Fiber: 5g; Sugar: 7g; Cholesterol: 0mg*

# Tofu, Chickpea, and Veggie Bowls

**DAIRY-FREE • GLUTEN-FREE • NUT-FREE • VEGETARIAN**
**Makes** 4 servings
**Prep time:** 30 minutes • **Cook time:** 45 minutes

Protein-packed with both tofu and chickpeas, this is a savory dish full of anti-inflammatory herbs like garlic, parsley, and ginger. Get creative with your ingredients and add as many veggies as you want! Consider broccoli, Brussels sprouts, cauliflower, mushrooms, green beans, cherry tomatoes, or bell peppers.

Garlic-Herb Marinated
  Tempeh or Tofu
  (page 95)
Basic Brown Rice
  (page 93)
Simple Ginger Teriyaki
  Sauce (page 90)
1 (15.5-ounce) can
  chickpeas, drained
  and rinsed
2 large carrots, shredded
2 cucumbers, chopped
1 cup chopped fresh
  parsley

1. Marinate the tofu and preheat the oven as directed in the tofu recipe.
2. Meanwhile, start the brown rice and make the teriyaki sauce as directed.
3. While the rice is simmering, transfer the tofu to the oven and finish cooking it.
4. Remove the brown rice from the heat.
5. If serving right away, in each of 4 bowls, create a base of brown rice. Top with the tofu, chickpeas, carrots, and cucumbers. Drizzle the bowls with the teriyaki sauce and garnish with parsley.
6. If storing for later, portion the tofu, rice, and beans together into 4 medium containers. Store the fresh vegetables and parsley separately in 4 small containers. Store the teriyaki sauce in a screw-top glass jar.

＊ **Storage:** Store all the components in the refrigerator for up to 5 days. To serve, microwave the tofu, rice, and beans for 1 to 2 minutes until heated through and follow the assembly instructions in step 5.

＊ **Cooking tip:** All of the vegetables in this recipe are raw, but if you prefer cooked vegetables, steam or roast the carrots for this bowl.

*Per Serving: Calories: 485; Total Fat: 15g; Saturated Fat: 2g; Protein: 22g; Total Carbohydrates: 68g; Fiber: 8g; Sugar: 13g; Cholesterol: 0mg*

# Almond Butter and Berry Sandwiches

**DAIRY-FREE · NIGHTSHADE-FREE · SOY-FREE · VEGAN**

**Makes** 5 sandwiches

**Prep time:** 5 minutes

A simple but sophisticated sandwich is a perfect meal-prep choice. Adults and kids alike will enjoy this healthy version of everyone's favorite comfort food, made entirely with anti-inflammatory ingredients. Serve with whole-grain crackers or chips, Edamame Hummus (page 153), or sliced raw vegetables, such as carrot sticks.

10 slices whole wheat or gluten-free bread

10 tablespoons natural almond butter (no added oil, sugar, or salt)

5 tablespoons no-sugar-added berry jam of your choice

10 large strawberries, thinly sliced

1. For each sandwich, lay 2 slices of bread on a flat surface. Spoon 2 tablespoons of almond butter on one of the slices and spread it to the edges. Top the almond butter with 1 tablespoon of berry jam and spread it. Add the sliced strawberries on top of the jam in a single layer. Top with the second piece of bread and cut in half on the diagonal.

2. Store the sandwiches in resealable plastic bags or storage containers. Keep all the remaining components portioned out for convenient use to make additional sandwiches.

\* **Storage:** A prepared sandwich will store well in the refrigerator for up to 2 days.

\* **Reuse tip:** Bread freezes well, so you can keep a loaf in the freezer and remove slices as you need them for meal prep.

*Per Serving (1 sandwich): Calories: 369; Total Fat: 20g; Saturated Fat: 2g; Protein: 15g; Total Carbohydrates: 36g; Fiber: 8g; Sugar: 6g; Cholesterol: 0mg*

# Black Bean and Mango Lettuce Wraps

**DAIRY-FREE • GLUTEN-FREE • NIGHTSHADE-FREE • NUT-FREE • SOY-FREE • VEGAN**

**Makes** 12 wraps (4 servings)

**Prep time:** 5 minutes • **Cook time:** 20 minutes

This simple wrap recipe is bold in both color and flavor, featuring anti-inflammatory black beans, mangos, cilantro, and lime. Garnished with rich Avocado Crema, these wraps are easy to assemble for a filling, protein-forward lunch. You'll likely have leftover lettuce from this recipe; use it to create a simple side to eat during the week.

Garlic-Lime Black Beans
  (page 155)
½ cup Avocado Crema
  (page 91)
1 head butter lettuce
1 teaspoon olive oil
Juice of 1 lime
¼ teaspoon salt
1 fresh mango, peeled
  and chopped, or
  1 cup thawed frozen
  mango chunks
2 scallions, thinly sliced
¾ cup chopped fresh
  cilantro

1. Cook the black beans as directed and set them aside to cool. While the beans cool, prepare the avocado crema as directed.
2. Remove 12 large, outer leaves of the lettuce to use as wraps.
3. In a medium bowl, whisk together the oil, lime juice, and salt. Add the mango, scallions, and cilantro and stir to combine.
4. If serving right away, put ⅓ cup of black bean mixture in the middle of each leaf of lettuce. Top with 1 to 2 tablespoons of the mango mixture and 1 to 2 teaspoons of avocado crema.
5. If storing for later, store the lettuce leaves, black beans, mango mixture, and avocado crema in separate storage containers.

✳ **Storage:** To serve, microwave the beans for 1 minute until heated through and follow assembly instructions in step 4.

✳ **Substitution tip:** Butter lettuce makes for great lettuce wraps because it's soft and pliable, but you can also use iceberg lettuce or romaine. Or skip the lettuce and make the wraps with corn tortillas.

*Per Serving (3 wraps): Calories: 379; Total Fat: 16g; Saturated Fat: 4g; Protein: 14g; Total Carbohydrates: 53g; Fiber: 17g; Sugar: 18g; Cholesterol: 0mg*

# Tempeh Wraps with Avocado and Veggies

**DAIRY-FREE • GLUTEN-FREE • NIGHTSHADE-FREE • NUT-FREE • VEGAN**
**Makes** 4 servings
**Prep time:** 10 minutes • **Cook time:** 20 minutes

A garlicky tempeh wrap with fresh veggies and creamy, anti-inflammatory avocado is the perfect lunch to keep you energized all afternoon long. Complemented with a homemade vegan Caesar dressing, this is a flavor-filled wrap that you'll make again and again.

Garlic-Herb Marinated
  Tempeh or Tofu
  (page 95)
Zesty Vegan Caesar
  Dressing (page 88)
4 large wraps or tortillas
  (whole wheat or corn, if
  you're gluten-free)
4 large romaine
  lettuce leaves
2 medium carrots, thinly
  sliced lengthwise
1 cup fresh sprouts (bean
  sprouts, radish, or
  broccoli sprouts)
2 avocados, sliced

1. Marinate and bake the tempeh as directed.
2. Meanwhile, make the dressing as directed.
3. If serving right away, for each wrap, lay a tortilla on a flat surface. Place a lettuce leaf on the tortilla, then spread ¼ cup of dressing on it with a spatula. Add one portion of carrot slices and ¼ cup of sprouts to each tortilla. Add 2 to 3 slices of tempeh, followed by half an avocado. Wrap the tortilla around the filling like a burrito, keeping the top open.
4. If storing for later, wrap the tortillas individually in plastic, then roll them in foil. Portion the tempeh, romaine, carrots, sprouts, and avocado halves into 4 large containers. Store the dressing in 4 individual small containers or a screw-top jar.

✱ **Storage:** Store all the components in the refrigerator. To serve, follow the assembly instructions in step 3. If you'd like, microwave the tempeh for 1 minute before adding it to the wrap.

✱ **Substitution tip:** Add other fresh veggies of your choice. If you eat nightshades, sliced raw bell peppers add flavor and crunch. You can also add thinly sliced cucumbers or raw zucchini.

*Per Serving: Calories: 597; Total Fat: 40g; Saturated Fat: 8g; Protein: 23g; Total Carbohydrates: 48g; Fiber: 15g; Sugar: 6g; Cholesterol: 0mg*

# Sweet Potato and Salmon Bowls

**DAIRY-FREE • GLUTEN-FREE • NIGHTSHADE-FREE • NUT-FREE • SOY-FREE**
**Makes** 4 servings
**Prep time:** 5 minutes • **Cook time:** 20 minutes

Vibrant sweet potatoes complement savory and salty salmon in this easy-to-assemble lunch bowl. You can make the sweet potatoes and salmon ahead of time, even baking them together in the oven, and then assemble the ingredients quickly and easily when you need a healthy, anti-inflammatory midday meal.

Fresh Dill Marinade
(page 87)

1 pound skin-on
salmon fillet

3 sweet potatoes,
peeled and cut into
¼-inch-thick rounds

3 tablespoons olive
oil, divided

½ teaspoon ground
cumin

½ teaspoon salt, divided

¼ teaspoon freshly
ground black
pepper, divided

2 large zucchini,
halved lengthwise
and cut crosswise
into half-moons

1. Preheat the oven to 400°F. Line 1 or 2 large sheet pans with parchment paper.
2. Prepare the dill marinade as directed and transfer it to a 9-by-12-inch glass baking dish.
3. Cut the salmon into four 4-ounce servings and place it flesh-side down in the marinade. Marinate for at least 20 minutes.
4. Meanwhile, arrange the sweet potato pieces on the pans. Drizzle with 2 tablespoons of olive oil and sprinkle with the cumin, ¼ teaspoon of salt, and ⅛ teaspoon of pepper. Bake them for 30 minutes, or until tender. Transfer to a wire cooling rack.
5. Replace the parchment paper on the sheet pans.
6. Place the zucchini on one side of the pan and the salmon pieces on the other side, skin-side down. Pour any remaining marinade on top of the salmon. Drizzle the zucchini with the remaining 1 tablespoon of olive oil and sprinkle with the remaining ¼ teaspoon of salt and ⅛ teaspoon of pepper. Bake for 14 to 18 minutes, until the salmon is just cooked through and the zucchini is golden brown. Cool before storing.
7. Portion the salmon, zucchini, and sweet potato slices into 4 large storage containers.

✳ **Storage:** Store in the refrigerator for up to 4 days. To serve, microwave for 1 to 2 minutes, until the ingredients are heated through. Transfer to a bowl to enjoy.

*Per Serving: Calories: 363; Total Fat: 18g; Saturated Fat: 3g; Protein: 26g; Total Carbohydrates: 25g; Fiber: 5g; Sugar: 8g; Cholesterol: 62mg*

Chipotle Chickpea Taco Bowls

*page 135*

CHAPTER

**9**

# Dinner

# Three-Bean Chili

**DAIRY-FREE • GLUTEN-FREE • NUT-FREE • SOY-FREE • VEGAN**
**Makes** 6 servings
**Prep time:** 20 minutes • **Cook time:** 30 minutes

Chili is the perfect meal-prep recipe. In this dish, kidney beans, white beans, and chickpeas offer a variety of anti-inflammatory fiber, vitamins, minerals, and antioxidants—no meat needed! The flavors in this dish mingle and develop with time; it may taste even better later in the week.

2 teaspoons olive oil
2 garlic cloves, minced
½ yellow onion, diced
2 green bell peppers, diced
1 (32-ounce) jar marinara sauce
2 cups corn kernels, canned, fresh, or frozen
1 (15.5-ounce) can red kidney beans, drained and rinsed
1 (15.5-ounce) can chickpeas, drained and rinsed
1 (15.5-ounce) can white beans (great northern or cannellini), drained and rinsed
1 cup water
1 teaspoon salt
1 teaspoon freshly ground black pepper
½ teaspoon chili powder
½ teaspoon dried oregano

1. In a large pot, heat the olive oil over medium heat. Add the garlic, onion, and bell peppers and sauté for 4 to 6 minutes, stirring occasionally, until the vegetables are soft and the onion becomes translucent.
2. Add the tomato sauce, corn, kidney beans, chickpeas, white beans, water, salt, black pepper, chili powder, and oregano. Increase the heat to high and bring the mixture to a boil, then reduce the heat to medium-low, cover, and simmer for 20 minutes. Add more water if needed to thin the chili to your preferred consistency. Cool before storing.
3. Portion the chili into 6 storage containers.

* **Storage:** Store the chili in the refrigerator for up to 5 days, or freeze it for up to 3 months. To serve, microwave for 2 minutes, stirring halfway through. Let frozen chili thaw overnight in the refrigerator before reheating.

* **Reuse tip:** This chili makes a large batch, so you can use it for lunches and dinners throughout the week (or even longer, if you freeze it). Garnish it with fresh cilantro or parsley, cheese (or nutritional yeast), or cubed avocado.

*Per Serving: Calories: 303; Total Fat: 4g; Saturated Fat: 1g; Protein: 16g; Total Carbohydrates: 57g; Fiber: 14g; Sugar: 9g; Cholesterol: 0mg*

# Turmeric-Ginger Chickpea Stew

**DAIRY-FREE • GLUTEN-FREE • NIGHTSHADE-FREE • NUT-FREE • SOY-FREE • VEGAN**

**Makes** 5 servings
**Prep time:** 15 minutes • **Cook time:** 45 minutes

Chickpeas provide a hearty base for this flavorful stew made with fresh, anti-inflammatory seasonings like turmeric, ginger, onion, and garlic. Coconut milk offers a creaminess that makes this stew rich and filling, without dairy. This recipe makes a large batch, so freeze what you won't eat within the week.

2 tablespoons olive oil

1 yellow onion, diced

2 garlic cloves, minced

1-inch piece fresh ginger, grated

1 teaspoon ground turmeric

1 (15.5-ounce) can chickpeas, drained and rinsed

½ teaspoon salt

1 teaspoon freshly ground black pepper

1 (15-ounce) can full-fat coconut milk

2 cups vegetable broth

1 bunch dinosaur/lacinato kale, stems and midribs removed, leaves chopped

1. In a large pot, heat the oil over medium heat. Add the onion and sauté for 2 to 4 minutes, stirring occasionally, until the onion has softened. Add the garlic and ginger and cook for 2 to 4 minutes more, stirring frequently, until fragrant. If the mixture is sticking to the pan, add a little water, 1 teaspoon at a time, and scrape up the stuck bits with a wooden spoon.

2. Add the turmeric, chickpeas, salt, and pepper and cook, stirring often, for 5 to 7 minutes, until the chickpeas start to brown and crisp slightly.

3. Add the coconut milk and broth. Bring the mixture to a simmer over medium-low heat and cook for 30 to 35 minutes, until the mixture has thickened and the chickpeas have absorbed the flavor of the herbs and spices.

4. Add the kale and cook until wilted and incorporated, 3 to 6 minutes. Cool the stew before storing.

5. Portion the stew into 6 storage containers.

* **Storage:** Store the stew in the refrigerator for up to 5 days, or freeze it for up to 3 months. To serve, microwave it for 1 to 2 minutes until heated through. Let frozen stew thaw overnight in the refrigerator before reheating.

* **Substitution tip:** Green cabbage, curly kale, Swiss chard, collard greens, or even spinach are easy substitutions for kale in this recipe. To add even more flavor, garnish with fresh mint, parsley, or basil leaves.

*Per Serving: Calories: 319; Total Fat: 25g; Saturated Fat: 17g; Protein: 7g; Total Carbohydrates: 22g; Fiber: 5g; Sugar: 5g; Cholesterol: 0mg*

# Lentil-Cauliflower Curry over Brown Rice

**DAIRY-FREE • GLUTEN-FREE • NIGHTSHADE-FREE • NUT-FREE • SOY-FREE • VEGAN**
**Makes** 5 servings
**Prep time:** 15 minutes • **Cook time:** 45 minutes

This hearty curry, made from protein-packed lentils and anti-inflammatory cauliflower, makes perfect leftovers, as its intense flavors continue to develop after it cooks. Fragrant curry powder, ground turmeric, and hearty vegetables create a savory base for this tasty, comforting dish.

Basic Brown Rice
   (page 93)
2 tablespoons coconut oil
1 yellow onion, diced
2 carrots, chopped
2 garlic cloves, minced
1 tablespoon curry
   powder (check label
   for nightshades)
1 teaspoon ground
   turmeric
½ teaspoon salt
½ teaspoon freshly
   ground black pepper
1 cup water, plus
   1 tablespoon
1½ cups brown
   lentils, rinsed
3 cups vegetable broth
1 small head cauliflower,
   chopped into florets
½ cup chopped fresh
   cilantro

1. Prepare the brown rice as directed.
2. Meanwhile, in a large skillet, heat the coconut oil over medium heat. Add the onion and carrots and sauté for 3 to 5 minutes, stirring occasionally, until the vegetables soften. Add the garlic and stir for 2 minutes, until fragrant. Add the curry powder, turmeric, salt, pepper, and 1 tablespoon of water and stir constantly for 2 minutes more.
3. Add the lentils and broth, cover, and simmer over medium heat for 30 minutes, until the lentils are soft and most of the water is absorbed.
4. Add the cauliflower and the remaining 1 cup of water, if needed to allow the cauliflower to cook. Cover the pot and simmer the curry for 7 to 8 minutes more, until the cauliflower has softened and can be pierced easily with a fork.
5. Remove the curry and brown rice from the heat and cool before storing.
6. Portion the lentil curry and rice side by side into 5 large storage containers. Store the cilantro separately in 5 small containers.

✱ **Storage:** Store in the refrigerator. To serve, microwave for 2 minutes, stirring after 1 minute. Garnish with cilantro.

*Per Serving: Calories: 509; Total Fat: 9g; Saturated Fat: 6g; Protein: 23g; Total Carbohydrates: 87g; Fiber: 12g; Sugar: 7g; Cholesterol: 0mg*

# Roasted Root Vegetables with Tempeh over Brown Rice

**DAIRY-FREE · GLUTEN-FREE · NIGHTSHADE-FREE · NUT-FREE · VEGAN**

**Makes** 5 servings

**Prep time:** 15 minutes · **Cook time:** 30 minutes

Garlicky marinated tempeh is the perfect protein to complement earthy, oven-roasted root vegetables. Served over simple brown rice, this meal will allow you to start incorporating naturally sweet vegetables into your diet—something kids and adults alike can enjoy.

Garlic-Herb Marinated
Tempeh or Tofu
(page 95)
Basic Brown Rice
(page 93)
1 large sweet potato,
peeled and chopped
2 carrots, halved
lengthwise, then
cut crosswise into
1-inch pieces
2 large golden beets,
washed, trimmed,
and chopped
1 red onion, cut into
large chunks
2 tablespoons olive oil
2 garlic cloves, minced
½ teaspoon salt
½ teaspoon freshly ground
black pepper
½ teaspoon ground
cinnamon

1. Preheat the oven to 400°F. Line a sheet pan with parchment paper.
2. Marinate the tempeh as directed and start the brown rice cooking.
3. Meanwhile, prep the sweet potato, carrots, beets, and onion and place them in a large bowl. Add the oil, garlic, salt, pepper, and cinnamon and stir to coat.
4. Pour the vegetables onto one half of the sheet pan. Roast the vegetables for 15 minutes, then remove the pan from the oven, flip the vegetables, and add the marinated tempeh to the other side of the pan. Drizzle the tempeh with any remaining marinade.
5. Roast the tempeh and vegetables for 15 minutes more, or until the vegetables are golden brown and can be pierced easily with a fork. Set aside to cool.
6. Once the brown rice is cooked, remove it from the heat and cool before storing.
7. Portion the rice, vegetables, and tempeh together in 5 large storage containers.

✳ **Storage:** Store in the refrigerator for up to 5 days. To serve, microwave the entire container for 2 minutes or until heated through. You can freeze the brown rice and tempeh for up to 2 months, but roasted vegetables won't thaw well—make a new batch when you need them.

*Per Serving: Calories: 387; Total Fat: 17g; Saturated Fat: 3g; Protein: 13g; Total Carbohydrates: 48g; Fiber: 4g; Sugar: 6g; Cholesterol: 0mg*

# Veggie Supreme Pan Pizza

**NUT-FREE • VEGETARIAN**

**Makes** 6 servings

**Prep time:** 15 minutes, plus 2 hours for the dough to rise • **Cook time:** 25 minutes

Pizza can be an anti-inflammatory food—if you make it the right way. A simple, whole-grain crust provides a nutrient- and fiber-rich base for a simple, healthy tomato sauce and an array of flavorful vegetables. If you don't want to make your own dough, see if your local grocery store sells premade dough in the refrigerated or freezer aisle.

---

**FOR THE PIZZA DOUGH**

1¼ cups warm (body temperature) water

1 envelope (2¼ teaspoons) rapid rise (fast-acting) yeast

¾ teaspoon sugar

1½ teaspoons salt

6 tablespoons olive oil, divided

1½ cups whole wheat flour

2½ cups unbleached all-purpose flour, divided, plus more for dusting

**FOR THE PIZZA**

2 tablespoons olive oil

2 garlic cloves, minced

1 (28-ounce) jar marinara sauce

1 teaspoon dried oregano

1 teaspoon dried basil

16 ounces shredded mozzarella cheese

8 ounces sliced mushrooms

2 cups arugula

1. Preheat the oven to 475°F.

**TO MAKE THE PIZZA DOUGH**

2. Pour the warm water into a small bowl or large glass measuring cup and add the yeast and sugar. Mix it together and let it stand for 3 to 5 minutes.

3. Transfer the yeast mixture to a large bowl or the bowl of a stand mixer and add the salt, 3 tablespoons of olive oil, the whole wheat flour, and 1½ cups of all-purpose flour. Beat in the remaining 1 cup of all-purpose flour, ¼ cup at a time, until the dough comes together enough to knead. Turn the dough out onto a floured surface and knead with your hands for about 5 minutes.

4. Spread the remaining 3 tablespoons of oil on a large sheet pan. Set the dough on the pan and cover it loosely with plastic wrap. Let it rise for 1 hour in a warm place.

**TO MAKE THE PIZZA**

5. Once the dough has risen, punch it down and form it into a rectangle the same size as the sheet pan. Gently prick the dough with a fork (so it doesn't bubble up in the oven), but don't poke through to the baking sheet. Cover the dough on the baking sheet with plastic wrap and let it rise for another hour.

6. Spread 2 tablespoons of oil onto the dough and sprinkle it with the garlic. Bake it in the oven for 5 minutes, until the garlic has started to brown and the dough has begun to cook.

7. Remove the partially baked crust from the oven and spread the marinara sauce over the entire surface of the crust, leaving a ½-inch border. Sprinkle with the oregano, basil, mozzarella, and mushrooms. Return the pizza to the oven and bake for 13 to 16 minutes more, until the crust has browned and the cheese is melted.

8. Sprinkle the pizza with fresh arugula and cut it into 12 slices.

9. Portion 2 slices into each of 6 large storage containers.

✳ **Storage:** Store the pizza in the refrigerator for up to 4 days, or freeze it for up to 2 months. To serve, microwave for 1 minute or reheat in the oven or toaster oven for 5 to 10 minutes at 350°F.

✳ **Substitution tip:** Try adding other toppings, like chopped bell peppers, pineapple, onion, or zucchini. You can also easily make this recipe dairy-free, gluten-free, or nightshade-free. Use a nondairy cheese, substitute gluten-free flour, or swap out the tomato sauce for additional olive oil.

*Per Serving:* Calories: 707; Total Fat: 36g; Saturated Fat: 13g; Protein: 27g; Total Carbohydrates: 68g; Fiber: 3g; Sugar: 2g; Cholesterol: 60mg

# Stuffed Portobello Mushrooms

**DAIRY-FREE • GLUTEN-FREE • NIGHTSHADE-FREE • NUT-FREE • SOY-FREE • VEGETARIAN**
**Makes** 4 servings
**Prep time:** 20 minutes • **Cook time:** 30 minutes

You'll be surprised at how savory and delicious portobello mushrooms can be when they serve as the vehicle for other anti-inflammatory elements like quinoa, onion, garlic, squash, and zucchini. These are healthy and create perfect leftovers to enjoy all week long.

Savory Herbed Quinoa
  (page 94)
Fresh Dill Marinade
  (page 87)
3 large portobello
  mushrooms,
  stems removed
1 tablespoon olive oil
½ yellow onion, diced
1 garlic clove, minced
1 cup cubed
  butternut squash
1 large zucchini, chopped
½ teaspoon salt
½ teaspoon freshly
  ground pepper
½ teaspoon
  ground cumin

1. Prepare the quinoa as directed.
2. Meanwhile, make the dill marinade as directed and place the mushrooms in it to marinate, gill-side down, for 10 minutes.
3. In a large skillet, heat the oil over medium heat. Add the onion, garlic, butternut squash, and zucchini and sauté for 6 to 8 minutes, until the vegetables are soft.
4. Preheat the oven to 400°F. Line a large sheet pan with parchment paper.
5. Once the quinoa is cooked and seasoned, add the butternut squash and zucchini mixture, salt, pepper, and cumin and stir to combine.
6. Set the same skillet used for the squash over medium heat. Add the mushrooms and 1 tablespoon of marinade, cover, and cook for 2 minutes on each side, until the mushrooms are softened slightly.
7. Transfer the mushrooms to the sheet pan, gill-side up and spoon ½ cup of quinoa filling into each mushroom (you'll have filling left over). Bake the mushrooms for 5 minutes and cool before storing.
8. Portion the stuffed mushrooms into 3 large storage containers. Top the containers with any remaining quinoa filling or freeze the extra filling separately.

✱ **Storage:** Store in the refrigerator for up to 3 days. To serve, microwave the mushrooms and quinoa filling for 1 to 2 minutes until heated through.

*Per Serving: Calories: 235; Total Fat: 9g; Saturated Fat: 2g; Protein: 9g; Total Carbohydrates: 33g; Fiber: 7g; Sugar: 7g; Cholesterol: 0mg*

# Lemon-Artichoke Risotto

**DAIRY-FREE • GLUTEN-FREE • NUT-FREE • SOY-FREE • VEGAN**
**Makes** 5 servings
**Prep time:** 15 minutes • **Cook time:** 40 minutes

This simple, meal prep-friendly risotto is a great way to enjoy a rich rice dish filled with anti-inflammatory herbs and vegetables, like delicate artichokes, bright lemon, and fragrant mint. This vegan recipe needs no dairy to achieve its creamy texture. For even more protein, add cooked chicken, shrimp, or tofu.

4 cups vegetable broth

4 tablespoons olive oil, divided

1 (14-ounce) can or jar artichoke hearts, drained and cut into quarters

4 ounces sugar snap peas, trimmed and cut in half

½ medium onion, diced

1½ cups Arborio rice

½ teaspoon salt

¼ cup chopped fresh chives

¼ cup chopped fresh mint

½ teaspoon freshly ground black pepper

Juice of ½ lemon

⅓ cup chopped fresh flat-leaf parsley

1. In a large pot, bring the broth to a low simmer over medium heat. Once it's warm, remove it from the heat and set aside.

2. Meanwhile, in a large skillet, heat 2 tablespoons of oil over medium heat. Add the artichoke hearts, snap peas, and onion and cook, stirring occasionally, for 6 to 8 minutes, until the artichoke has begun to brown and the onion is soft and translucent. Transfer the mixture to a small bowl and set aside.

3. In the same skillet, heat the remaining 2 tablespoons of oil over medium heat. Add the rice and salt and stir to coat the rice. Cook the mixture for 2 to 3 minutes, stirring constantly—the rice may start to sizzle or crackle. Reduce the heat to medium-low, then add the broth 1 cup at a time, stirring after each cup until the liquid is absorbed (5 to 8 minutes per cup). Continue stirring so that the risotto becomes thick and creamy, 20 to 30 minutes total. Taste the risotto to ensure the grains are not too firm, and if it needs to cook longer, add up to 1 cup of water, ⅓ cup at a time, and stir until the liquid absorbs.

# Lemon-Artichoke Risotto

*Continued*

4. Once the risotto is finished cooking and the liquid is absorbed, stir in the chives, mint, pepper, and the artichoke heart mixture. Once that's incorporated into the mixture, add the lemon juice and parsley.
5. Portion the risotto into 5 medium storage containers.

✳ **Storage:** Store the risotto in the refrigerator, or freeze it for up to 3 months. To serve, reheat in the microwave for 1 to 2 minutes and stir. For frozen risotto, thaw in the refrigerator overnight before reheating.

✳ **Substitution tip:** Add different herbs to switch things up—swap chives for scallions, use fresh basil instead of mint, or try cilantro instead of parsley. Dried herbs can be substituted for fresh ones. Use 1 teaspoon each of basil and parsley. If you don't have fresh snap peas, you can add ½ cup of frozen peas instead.

*Per Serving: Calories: 430; Total Fat: 14g; Saturated Fat: 2g; Protein: 7g; Total Carbohydrates: 68g; Fiber: 6g; Sugar: 3g; Cholesterol: 0mg*

# Chipotle Chickpea Taco Bowls

**DAIRY-FREE • GLUTEN-FREE • NUT-FREE • SOY-FREE • VEGAN**
**Makes** 4 servings
**Prep time:** 10 minutes • **Cook time:** 10 minutes

No tortillas are needed for this filling taco bowl recipe, packed with seasoned chickpeas, savory black beans, zesty greens, and creamy avocado. The recipe is easy to adapt—add or remove toppings based on whatever you feel like having on any given day. The "taco seasoning" is an easy anti-inflammatory spice blend you can make in minutes.

Garlic-Lime Black Beans
(page 155)
Avocado Crema
(page 91)
⅓ cup Anti-Inflammatory
Multiuse Spice Blend
(page 84)
1 tablespoon olive oil
½ yellow onion, diced
½ tablespoon
chipotle chile
powder, or 1 canned
chipotle pepper in
adobo, chopped
1 tablespoon water
2 (15.5-ounce) cans
chickpeas, drained
and rinsed
4 cups arugula
2 cups halved cherry
tomatoes
1 large avocado, sliced
or diced

1. Prepare the black beans as directed.
2. While the beans cook, prepare the avocado crema and spice blend as directed.
3. In a large skillet, heat the oil over medium heat. Add the onion and sauté for 2 to 4 minutes, stirring occasionally, until softened. Add the chipotle, spice blend, and water and stir to cook until the mixture is fragrant, 2 minutes more. Add the chickpeas and cook for 2 to 4 minutes more, until the chickpeas are incorporated into the mixture and heated through.
4. If serving right away, fill 4 bowls each with 1 cup of arugula, then top them with single portions of the chipotle chickpeas, black beans, ½ cup of cherry tomatoes, and one-quarter of the avocado. Drizzle with avocado crema.
5. If storing for later, portion the chipotle chickpeas and black beans together into 4 medium storage containers. Store the arugula in 4 large containers along with one-quarter of the avocado and ½ cup of cherry tomatoes. Store the avocado crema in 4 small containers.

✳ **Storage:** To serve, microwave the chickpeas and beans for 1 to 2 minutes and follow the assembly instructions in step 4.

✳ **Substitution tip:** Make these bowls your own by changing ingredients to switch up the flavor. Try adding corn, tortilla strips, cheese, chopped tomato, bell pepper, cucumber, or salsa.

*Per Serving: Calories: 634; Total Fat: 29g; Saturated Fat: 6g; Protein: 25g; Total Carbohydrates: 78g; Fiber: 28g; Sugar: 13g; Cholesterol: 0mg*

# Creamy Avocado Vegetable Burritos

**DAIRY-FREE • NIGHTSHADE-FREE • NUT-FREE • SOY-FREE • VEGAN**

**Makes** 4 servings

**Prep time:** 10 minutes • **Cook time:** 10 minutes

Burritos are the ultimate meal-prep recipe. When wrapped in foil, they stay fresh in the refrigerator for a couple of days and are easy to reheat in a minute or two. They freeze well, too. These burritos have a base of protein- and fiber-packed pinto beans. A variety of veggies add color, flavor, and anti-inflammatory vitamins and antioxidants. The best part about this recipe, though? Lots and lots of avocado.

Avocado Crema
  (page 91)
1 tablespoon olive oil
1 yellow onion,
  thinly sliced
1 zucchini, diced
½ teaspoon salt
½ teaspoon freshly
  ground pepper
½ teaspoon
  ground cumin
1 (15.5-ounce) can
  pinto beans, drained
  and rinsed
½ small head
  cabbage, shredded
4 large tortillas, whole
  wheat or gluten-free
½ cup chopped
  fresh cilantro
1 large avocado, sliced

1. Make the avocado crema as directed.
2. In a large skillet, heat the oil over medium heat. Add the onion and zucchini, stirring occasionally for 5 to 7 minutes, until the vegetables soften. Add the salt, pepper, cumin, and beans and stir well to combine, cooking 1 to 2 minutes more, until the bean filling is hot.
3. In a large bowl, combine the cabbage and avocado crema and stir to combine.
4. Assemble as many burritos as you will eat in 2 days. For each burrito, lay a tortilla on a flat surface and top with one-quarter of the bean filling, followed by one-quarter of the cabbage and crema mixture. Sprinkle with the cilantro and add one-quarter of the avocado on top. Wrap the burrito tightly by folding down the top and bottom of the tortilla over the filling, and wrapping the left and right sides so they overlap.

**5.** Wrap the assembled burritos individually in foil and refrigerate. For the remaining components, portion the bean mixture evenly into medium containers, and store the cabbage and crema mixture, avocado, and cilantro in separate small containers. Store the tortillas individually rolled in paper towel and foil.

✳ **Storage:** Store premade burritos in the refrigerator for up to 2 days. To serve, pop them in the oven at 350°F for 10 to 15 minutes or remove them from the foil, wrap them in a paper towel, and microwave briefly. To make more burritos from the stored components, microwave the bean mixture for 1 to 2 minutes, or until heated through. Heat the tortilla for 10 to 20 seconds until soft. Assemble and wrap the burritos per step 4.

✳ **Substitution tip:** Spice these burritos up with salsa or hot sauce. Or try making them "wet" burritos by smothering them with Homemade Enchilada Sauce (page 92)—you'll need 2 cups for 4 burritos.

*Per Serving: Calories: 516; Total Fat: 26g; Saturated Fat: 7g; Protein: 15g; Total Carbohydrates: 63g; Fiber: 19g; Sugar: 11g; Cholesterol: 0mg*

# Shrimp Pasta Bake with Fresh Greens

**DAIRY-FREE • NIGHTSHADE-FREE • NUT-FREE • SOY-FREE**
**Makes** 4 servings
**Prep time:** 15 minutes • **Cook time:** 10 minutes

This is an anti-inflammatory spin on a classic comfort meal. Once you get this in the oven, it's hands-off, making it perfect for multitasking and meal prep. You'll love the zesty, lemony shrimp cooked with fragrant, anti-inflammatory herbs. Try this dish sprinkled with Parmesan cheese or nutritional yeast for added flavor.

3 tablespoons olive oil, divided

1 pound frozen peeled cooked large or medium shrimp, thawed

16 ounces whole wheat or bean/lentil fusilli pasta

3 garlic cloves, minced

½ yellow onion, diced

1 teaspoon dried basil

1 teaspoon dried oregano

1 teaspoon dried thyme

½ teaspoon salt

½ teaspoon freshly ground black pepper

Juice of 1 lemon

8 cups salad greens

1. Preheat the oven to 350°F. Grease a 9-by-13-inch glass baking dish with 1 tablespoon of olive oil.

2. Make sure the shrimp are thawed completely. Rinse them with cold water and pat dry with a paper towel. Set aside on a plate.

3. Bring a large pot of water to a boil over high heat. Add the pasta and cook according to the package directions. Drain and transfer to a large bowl.

4. While the pasta is cooking, in a large skillet, heat the remaining 2 tablespoons of oil over medium heat. Add the garlic and onion and cook for 3 to 4 minutes, until the onion is soft and translucent. Add the shrimp and sprinkle evenly with the basil, oregano, thyme, salt, and pepper. Heat the shrimp, stirring them to encourage even heating, for 2 to 3 minutes. Remove from the heat and add the lemon juice.

5. Pour the shrimp mixture over the pasta and stir it to incorporate. Transfer the entire mixture to the prepared baking dish and bake for 25 to 30 minutes, until lightly browned on top. Cool before storing.

**6.** Divide the pasta bake among 4 medium storage containers. Place 2 cups of the greens into each of 4 large containers.

✳ **Storage:** Store in the refrigerator for 3 to 4 days. To serve, microwave the pasta for 1 to 2 minutes until heated through, then pour it over the salad greens.

✳ **Ingredient tip:** Thaw shrimp in a bowl of cold water in the refrigerator. If using uncooked shrimp, cook them in step 4 for 4 minutes on one side and 2 minutes on the other, until they are pink and no longer translucent. If you can't find peeled cooked shrimp, peel them after thawing.

*Per Serving: Calories: 624; Total Fat: 13g; Saturated Fat: 2g; Protein: 39g; Total Carbohydrates: 90g; Fiber: 5g; Sugar: 5g; Cholesterol: 183mg*

# Sheet Pan Salmon and Asparagus with Roasted Potatoes

**DAIRY-FREE • GLUTEN-FREE • NUT-FREE • SOY-FREE**
**Makes** 4 servings
**Prep time:** 20 minutes • **Cook time:** 1 hour

This simple sheet pan meal is a balance of heart-healthy complex carbohydrates, omega-3-packed protein, and fiber-rich, antioxidant-filled vegetables. The recipe also uses fresh, savory herbs for more flavor and health benefits. Make your meal-prep days easy and fun with this hands-off recipe that allows you to multitask in the kitchen.

Roasted Red Potatoes
   with Herbs (page 154)
Fresh Dill Marinade
   (page 87), divided
1 pound skin-on
   salmon fillet
2 bunches asparagus,
   woody ends
   snapped off

1. Preheat the oven to 400°F.
2. Prepare the potatoes as directed and put them in the oven.
3. Make the dill marinade as directed. Measure out ⅓ cup and set it aside. Transfer the remaining ⅔ cup of marinade to a glass baking dish.
4. Cut the salmon into four 4-ounce servings and place it flesh-side down in the baking dish. Marinate for 20 minutes.
5. Cut the asparagus spears in half and place them in a large bowl. Add the reserved ⅓ cup of marinade and toss to coat.
6. Once the potatoes have been cooking for 40 minutes, remove the pan from the oven, flip the potatoes, and push them to one side of the pan. Place the salmon in the middle of the pan, skin-side down, and the asparagus on the other side. Drizzle the salmon and asparagus with any remaining marinade.
7. Bake for 15 to 20 minutes more, until the asparagus is slightly browned and the salmon is just cooked through. Let cool before storing.
8. Evenly portion the potatoes, salmon, and asparagus into 4 large containers, placing the salmon in the middle.

✳ **Storage:** Store in the refrigerator for up to 4 days. To serve, reheat the container in the microwave for 1 to 2 minutes, until heated through.

*Per Serving: Calories: 377; Total Fat: 14g; Saturated Fat: 2g; Protein: 28g; Total Carbohydrates: 35g; Fiber: 7g; Sugar: 5g; Cholesterol: 62mg*

# Baked Salmon Cakes

**DAIRY-FREE • NIGHTSHADE-FREE • NUT-FREE • SOY-FREE**
**Makes** 8 salmon cakes (4 servings)
**Prep time:** 25 minutes • **Cook time:** 20 minutes

Using leftover salmon or canned salmon can help cut down on food waste, and that's where this recipe comes in. These simple, hands-off salmon cakes are baked rather than fried and are full of anti-inflammatory benefits thanks to the omega-3 fatty acids in the salmon. The health benefits get a boost by being served on a bed of romaine with avocado dressing.

2 (5-ounce) cans salmon or 10 ounces leftover cooked salmon
1 large egg, beaten
1 tablespoon grapeseed or avocado oil
2 scallions, chopped
¼ cup chopped fresh parsley
2 cups whole wheat or gluten-free bread crumbs, divided
Juice of ½ large lemon
1 tablespoon Dijon mustard
1 teaspoon salt
1 teaspoon freshly ground black pepper
¼ teaspoon onion powder
Double batch Creamy Avocado Dressing (page 89)
6 cups chopped romaine lettuce

1. Preheat the oven to 375°F. Line a sheet pan with parchment paper.
2. In a large bowl, combine the salmon, egg, oil, scallions, parsley, 1 cup of bread crumbs, the lemon juice, mustard, salt, pepper, and onion powder and stir well to combine. Use your hands to form the mixture into 8 round patties of equal size.
3. Pour the remaining 1 cup of bread crumbs onto a plate and dip the patties in the bread crumbs to coat on all sides. Arrange the breaded salmon cakes in a single layer on the sheet pan.
4. Bake for 15 to 20 minutes, flipping halfway through, until golden brown on both sides. Let cool before storing.
5. While the salmon cakes are baking, make the avocado dressing as directed.
6. Place 2 salmon cakes in each of 4 medium storage containers. Divide the lettuce evenly into 4 medium containers. Portion the avocado dressing evenly into 4 small containers.

✳ **Storage:** Store the salmon cakes in the refrigerator for up to 4 days. They can be frozen for up to 3 months. To serve, microwave the salmon cakes for 1 to 2 minutes (thaw first if frozen). Pour the dressing on the lettuce and top with hot salmon cakes.

✳ **Substitution tip:** Use this same recipe to make crab cakes. Use 10 ounces of lump crabmeat (picked over to remove bits of shell); the assembly and cooking are the same.

*Per Serving (2 salmon cakes): Calories: 569; Total Fat: 29g; Saturated Fat: 6g; Protein: 25g; Total Carbohydrates: 57g; Fiber: 12g; Sugar: 11g; Cholesterol: 94mg*

# Fish Tacos with Cabbage Slaw

**DAIRY-FREE • GLUTEN-FREE • NIGHTSHADE-FREE • NUT-FREE • SOY-FREE**
**Makes** 8 tacos (4 servings)
**Prep time:** 20 minutes • **Cook time:** 8 minutes

Use whatever type of fish you like best in these tacos—or for a vegan or vegetarian option, use tofu or tempeh instead, preparing it as you would the fish. These tacos are topped with healthy cabbage slaw and served with a side of garlicky black beans.

Double batch
  Honey-Lime Vinaigrette
  with Fresh Herbs
  (page 85), divided
1 pound cod, red snapper,
  or halibut
1 small head green
  cabbage, shredded
1 large carrot, shredded
Garlic-Lime Black Beans
  (page 155)
¼ cup grapeseed
  or avocado oil
8 (6-inch) corn tortillas
½ cup chopped
  fresh cilantro

1. Prepare the vinaigrette as directed and pour 1 cup of it into a glass baking dish. Place the fish into the marinade, flesh-side down, and set it aside to marinate for at least 20 minutes.
2. Meanwhile, in a large bowl, combine the cabbage and carrots. Pour in the remaining 1 cup vinaigrette and toss to coat. Set the slaw aside.
3. Prepare the black beans as directed and set aside.
4. In a large skillet, heat the oil over medium-high heat. Add the fish and cook on one side for 4 minutes. Flip the fish and cook the other side for at least 1 minute, until the fish is cooked through. Slice the fish into 8 equal portions (about 2 ounces each).
5. If serving right away, heat the tortillas and place one portion of fish onto each tortilla. Top the fish with about ⅓ cup of cabbage slaw. Sprinkle with the cilantro. Serve a portion of black beans on the side.
6. If storing for later, store 4 sets of 2 tortillas each rolled up in plastic wrap and then foil. Portion two 2-ounce servings of fish and one ½-cup serving of beans into each of 4 medium containers. Divide the cabbage slaw and cilantro equally among 4 medium containers.

✱ **Storage:** Store all the components in the refrigerator for up to 4 days. To serve, microwave the fish and beans for 1 minute. Microwave the tortillas for 20 seconds. Follow the assembly instructions in step 5.

***Per Serving (2 tacos):*** *Calories: 634; Total Fat: 18g; Saturated Fat: 2g; Protein: 32g; Total Carbohydrates: 88g; Fiber: 19g; Sugar: 27g; Cholesterol: 53mg*

# Easy Bean Veggie Burgers

**DAIRY-FREE • NIGHTSHADE-FREE • NUT-FREE • SOY-FREE • VEGETARIAN**
**Makes** 6 servings
**Prep time:** 10 minutes • **Cook time:** 20 minutes

Store-bought veggie burgers can be a challenge. Many are heavily processed. Others contain mostly grains and very little protein, which can leave you feeling hungry again soon after eating. These bean and veggie burgers are simple to make, they freeze and reheat well, and they're delicious and savory—no meat required!

1 (15.5-ounce) can
   black beans, drained
   and rinsed
1 (15.5-ounce) can
   chickpeas, drained
   and rinsed
½ yellow onion, diced
3 garlic cloves, minced
2 large eggs
1 teaspoon ground cumin
¾ teaspoon salt
¾ teaspoon freshly
   ground black pepper
1 cup whole wheat
   or gluten-free
   bread crumbs
½ cup old-fashioned
   rolled oats
6 whole wheat
   or gluten-free
   hamburger buns
2 avocados
6 large romaine
   lettuce leaves

1. Preheat the oven to 375°F. Line a sheet pan with parchment paper.
2. In a large bowl, mash the black beans and chickpeas with a fork or potato masher until they form a thick paste. If you'd like, leave some whole or partially whole beans for texture. Add the onion and garlic and stir to incorporate.
3. In a small bowl, whisk together the eggs, cumin, salt, and pepper. Pour it over the bean mixture and stir to combine. Stir in the bread crumbs and oats (the mixture should be somewhat sticky and hold together when pressed). Divide the mixture into 6 portions and use your hands to shape them into round patties.
4. Arrange the patties in a single layer on the sheet pan. Bake for 30 minutes, flipping halfway through, until slightly crispy on the edges. Cool before storing or freezing.

*Continued* ❯

# Easy Bean Veggie Burgers

*Continued*

5. If serving right away, split and toast the buns for 2 to 3 minutes. Place a patty on the bun and smear one-third of an avocado on the top of the burger. Top with a large romaine leaf.
6. If storing for later, place 1 burger in each of 6 medium containers. Divide the 2 avocados each into thirds (you should have 6 sections total). Store the avocado, lettuce, and buns in individual containers or resealable bags.

✻ **Storage:** Store all the components in the refrigerator. The patties can be frozen for up to 3 months. To serve, microwave the patty for 1 to 2 minutes (thaw first if frozen). Follow the assembly instructions in step 5.

✻ **Cooking tip:** You can also cook these patties in a large skillet over medium-high heat. Use 2 tablespoons of olive oil and cook the patties for 6 minutes on each side. Add other toppings such as barbecue sauce, mustard, ketchup, hot sauce, spinach, or tomato slices.

*Per Serving: Calories: 515; Total Fat: 17g; Saturated Fat: 3g; Protein: 21g; Total Carbohydrates: 74g; Fiber: 18g; Sugar: 10g; Cholesterol: 62mg*

Fruit and Herb Salad Parfaits
*page 99*

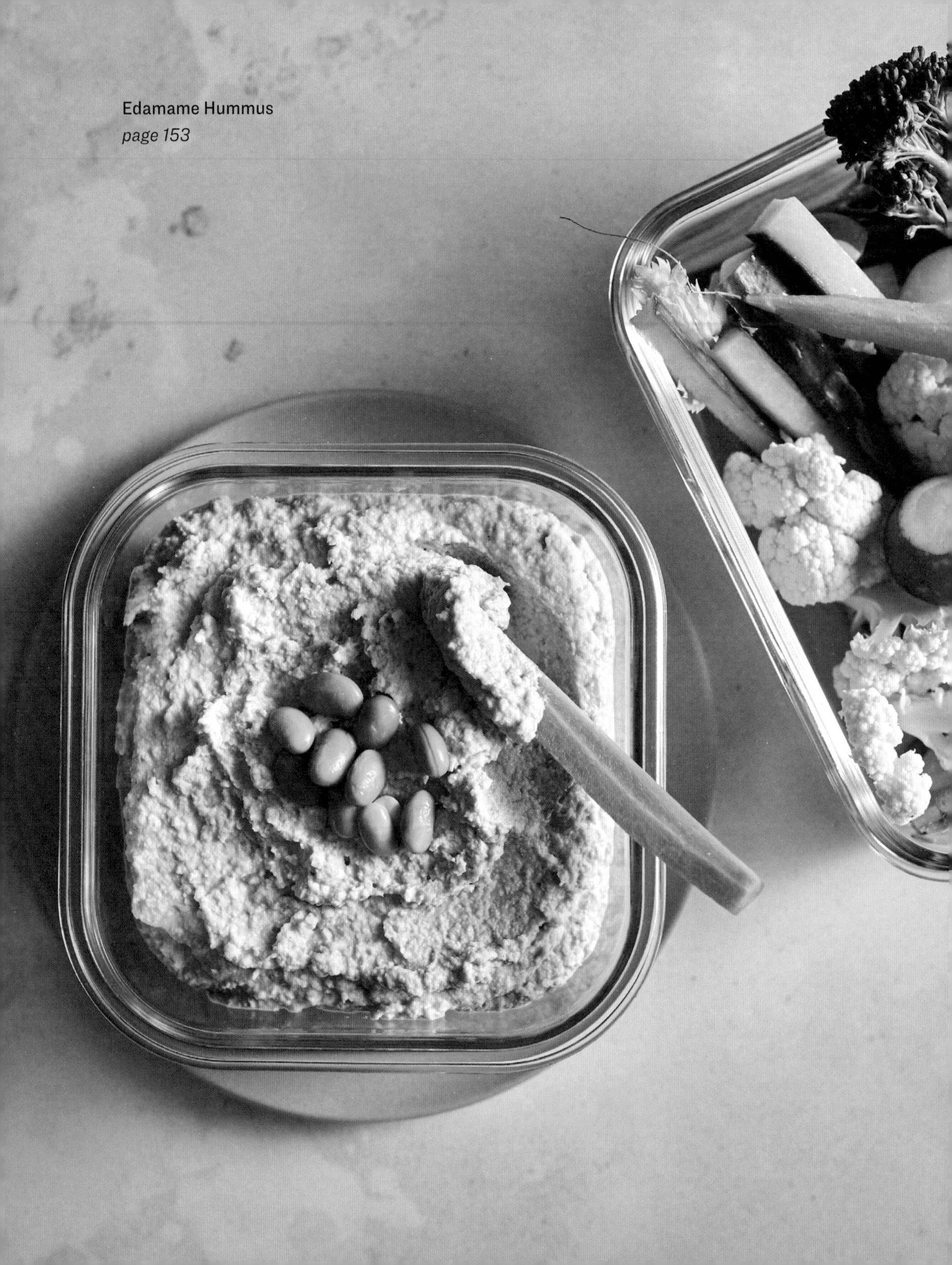

Edamame Hummus

*page 153*

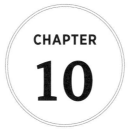

CHAPTER

# 10

# Snacks and Sides

# Turmeric Golden Milk Tea

**DAIRY-FREE • GLUTEN-FREE • NIGHTSHADE-FREE • NUT-FREE • SOY-FREE • VEGETARIAN**
**Makes** 5 servings
**Prep time:** 10 minutes • **Cook time:** 5 minutes

Sometimes, between meals, you want a warm, comforting, and slightly sweet snack that's also healthy and anti-inflammatory. Snacks should provide your body with a balance of protein, carbohydrates, and fat for sustained energy. Next time you find yourself craving something warm, savory, and sweet, whip up a simple mug of this to sip on.

2 cups boiling water

3 ginger tea bags

3 cups unsweetened oat milk, warmed

1 teaspoon ground cinnamon

1½ teaspoons ground turmeric

1 teaspoon ground ginger

2 teaspoons honey

1. In a large glass measuring cup or medium bowl, pour the boiling water over the tea bags. Steep for 5 minutes. Remove the tea bags and add the warmed oat milk, cinnamon, turmeric, ginger, and honey.
2. Transfer the mixture to a blender and blend until frothy, about 20 seconds. Cool before storing.
3. Divide the golden milk tea equally among 5 glass mason jars.

✳ **Storage:** Store in the refrigerator for up to 1 week. Or portion into individual 1-cup servings and freeze for up to 2 months. To serve, reheat refrigerated or frozen golden milk in the microwave or on the stovetop. Sprinkle the hot milk tea with more cinnamon, if desired.

✳ **Substitution tip:** For a milder flavor, reduce the cinnamon and ginger. Try using other types of unsweetened nondairy milk, such as soy, rice, almond, cashew, or coconut, but keep in mind this will change the calories, protein, and fat content of the recipe.

*Per Serving: Calories: 93; Total Fat: 3g; Saturated Fat: 0g; Protein: 5g; Total Carbohydrates: 13g; Fiber: 1g; Sugar: 8g; Cholesterol: 0mg*

# Banana Energy Cookies

**DAIRY-FREE • GLUTEN-FREE • NIGHTSHADE-FREE • NUT-FREE • SOY-FREE • VEGAN**
**Makes** 8 cookies (4 servings)
**Prep time:** 5 minutes • **Cook time:** 20 minutes

Cookies don't have to be packed with butter and sugar—they can be naturally sweet and satisfying and still healthy. These two-ingredient cookies are quick and easy snacks. They freeze well and, of course, are made only with anti-inflammatory ingredients.

1 cup old-fashioned rolled oats

1½ large very ripe bananas, mashed

Optional: ½ cup mix-ins of choice, such as chopped walnuts, chocolate chips, or dried cranberries, or 1 teaspoon cinnamon or pure vanilla extract

1. Preheat the oven to 350°F. Line a baking sheet with parchment paper.
2. In a large bowl, combine the oats and mashed banana. Mix with a wooden spoon until the oats are thoroughly coated and a crumbly dough forms. Add any mix-ins and stir to combine.
3. Scoop out spoonfuls of dough and use your fingers to press the dough together to form eight 1½-inch cookies. Place the dough balls 2 inches apart on the baking sheet and press slightly to flatten.
4. Bake the cookies for 20 minutes, or until lightly browned. Set aside to cool.
5. Store the cooled cookies in a storage container.

✳ **Storage:** Store in the refrigerator for up to 5 days. To freeze, store in a freezer bag for up to 3 months.

✳ **Cooking tip:** The cookie dough may be on the wetter side if you use larger bananas. If the dough is too wet, add more oats ⅛ cup at a time until a crumbly dough forms.

*Per Serving (2 cookies): Calories: 197; Total Fat: 3g; Saturated Fat: 0g; Protein: 7g; Total Carbohydrates: 37g; Fiber: 6g; Sugar: 6g; Cholesterol: 0mg*

# Chocolate Chia Seed Pudding

**DAIRY-FREE • GLUTEN-FREE • NIGHTSHADE-FREE • NUT-FREE • VEGAN**

**Makes** 5 servings
**Prep time:** 5 minutes, plus 5 hours to chill

This decadent chia seed pudding makes a nice treat, snack, or dessert any time of day. Naturally sweetened with just a touch of maple syrup, this recipe is high in fiber and anti-inflammatory omega-3 fatty acids, thanks to the chia seeds. It's also antioxidant-rich thanks to the cocoa! Feel free to adjust the amount of maple syrup to your preferred sweetness.

2 tablespoons unsweetened cocoa powder

2 tablespoons maple syrup

1 teaspoon pure vanilla extract

1½ cups unsweetened soy or oat milk

½ cup chia seeds

1. In a medium bowl, combine the cocoa, maple syrup, vanilla, milk, and chia seeds and whisk to combine. The cocoa may take 1 to 2 minutes to incorporate; keep whisking until no lumps remain.
2. Cover the bowl and refrigerate it for 30 minutes.
3. Remove the bowl from the refrigerator and stir the mixture. Refrigerate it again for another 30 minutes and then stir it again, to ensure the mixture sets evenly. Leave the bowl in the refrigerator for 4 or more hours, until the mixture has a thick, pudding-like consistency.
4. Divide the pudding into 5 storage containers or screw-top jars.

\* **Storage:** Store the pudding in the refrigerator for up to 5 days, or freeze it for up to 2 months. If frozen, thaw in the refrigerator for 3 to 5 hours before serving. If the pudding has become too thick, stir in 1 to 2 teaspoons of milk to thin as needed.

\* **Reuse tip:** Get creative with toppings! Try adding chopped berries, banana slices, coconut flakes, or chopped nuts.

*Per Serving: Calories: 178; Total Fat: 9g; Saturated Fat: 1g; Protein: 7g; Total Carbohydrates: 21g; Fiber: 9g; Sugar: 8g; Cholesterol: 0mg*

# Homemade Fruit and Nut Granola Bars

**DAIRY-FREE • GLUTEN-FREE • NIGHTSHADE-FREE • SOY-FREE • VEGAN**
**Makes** 8 granola bars
**Prep time:** 10 minutes, plus 2 hours to chill

Once you discover how easy it is to make your own granola bars—eliminating the added sugars and oils in store-bought brands—you'll find yourself making these a part of every meal-prep day. These bars set in the refrigerator, so they're perfect to meal prep and eat for breakfast or a snack all week long.

1 teaspoon coconut oil

1 cup chopped pitted
  Medjool dates
  (6 large dates)

½ cup almond butter

½ cup hulled
  pumpkin seeds

½ cup slivered almonds

1 cup dried fruit, such
  as raisins, cranberries,
  or cherries

1 teaspoon ground
  cinnamon

2 tablespoons water

1. Grease an 8-by-8-inch glass baking dish with the coconut oil. Line it with parchment paper so that the parchment paper comes all the way up the sides of the dish.

2. In a food processor, combine the dates, almond butter, pumpkin seeds, almonds, dried fruit, cinnamon, and water and pulse the mixture until just combined, but not completely blended. The dough should be cohesive but textured and crumbly. If the dough is not blending, push it around the food processor with a spoon or add more water 1 tablespoon at a time, pulsing in between.

3. Form the dough loosely into a ball and transfer it to the lined baking dish. With your hands, press it into the pan to make it even (about 1½ inches thick) and so it reaches into the corners.

4. Refrigerate the dough for 1 to 2 hours, then remove it from the refrigerator and grab the edges of the parchment paper to lift it out of the baking dish. Place the granola on a cutting board and use a sharp knife to cut it into 8 bars.

5. Transfer the bars to a storage container.

✳ **Storage:** Store in the refrigerator for up to 7 days.

✳ **Substitution tip:** Try using different types of nut or seed butters instead of almond, such as peanut butter or tahini. When reading labels, look for nut butters that don't have added oils or sugar.

***Per Serving (1 granola bar):*** *Calories: 289; Total Fat: 16g; Saturated Fat: 2g; Protein: 8g; Total Carbohydrates: 34g; Fiber: 5g; Sugar: 24g; Cholesterol: 0mg*

# Simple Garlic-Roasted Chickpeas

**DAIRY-FREE • GLUTEN-FREE • NIGHTSHADE-FREE • NUT-FREE • SOY-FREE • VEGAN**
**Makes** 5 servings
**Prep time:** 10 minutes • **Cook time:** 25 minutes

Roasted chickpeas make the perfect high-fiber, high-protein, anti-inflammatory snack. Perfect for kids and adults alike, this savory, crunchy grab-and-go snack can be portioned into small containers or bags to enjoy when a craving hits.

1 (15.5-ounce) can
  chickpeas, drained
  and rinsed
1½ tablespoons olive oil
2 garlic cloves, minced
½ teaspoon dried
  oregano
½ teaspoon dried thyme
½ teaspoon salt
½ teaspoon freshly
  ground black pepper

1. Preheat the oven to 400°F. Line a large sheet pan with parchment paper.
2. Spread the rinsed chickpeas on a clean kitchen towel and use another towel to pat them dry.
3. Transfer the chickpeas to a large bowl and drizzle them with the oil. Add the garlic, oregano, thyme, salt, and pepper. Toss the mixture to coat the chickpeas.
4. Transfer the chickpeas to the sheet pan and bake them for 10 minutes. Flip them with a spatula and bake them for 10 to 15 minutes more, until they're golden brown. Check them frequently during the last 5 minutes to avoid burning. Cool before storing.
5. Transfer the cooled chickpeas to small jars, resealable bags, or storage containers.

✳ **Storage:** Store at room temperature for up to 3 days. The chickpeas may start to lose their crunchy texture after the second day, but they're still delicious! Feel free to crisp them back up for 3 to 5 minutes in the toaster oven.

✳ **Substitution tip:** Get creative adding new spices or adjusting spice levels to taste. Consider swapping in cumin, turmeric, curry, paprika, or even chili powder.

*Per Serving: Calories: 119; Total Fat: 5g; Saturated Fat: 1g; Protein: 4g; Total Carbohydrates: 14g; Fiber: 4g; Sugar: 2g; Cholesterol: 0mg*

# Edamame Hummus

**DAIRY-FREE • GLUTEN-FREE • NIGHTSHADE-FREE • NUT-FREE • VEGAN**

**Makes** 5 servings

**Prep time:** 10 minutes • **Cook time:** 5 minutes

Edamame hummus is the perfect way to boost protein and antioxidants in dip form. This hummus tastes great on whole-grain crackers, chips, and fresh veggies, like carrots, bell peppers, cucumber, tomatoes, broccoli, cauliflower, or celery. This recipe uses frozen edamame, so you can make it even if you don't have fresh edamame on hand.

8 ounces frozen shelled edamame

¼ cup tahini

Juice of 1 large lemon

1 garlic clove, halved

¾ teaspoon salt

½ teaspoon ground cumin

2 to 4 tablespoons water

3 tablespoons olive oil

1. Microwave the frozen edamame for 2 to 3 minutes, or per package instructions.
2. In a food processor or blender, combine the edamame, tahini, lemon juice, garlic, salt, cumin, and 2 tablespoons of water. Puree the mixture until it's smooth. If it needs more liquid, add up to 2 more tablespoons of water, 1 tablespoon at a time. With the food processor running, slowly drizzle in the olive oil 1 tablespoon at a time, blending well to incorporate after each addition.
3. Portion the hummus into 5 small storage containers.

✳ **Storage:** Store in the refrigerator for up to 7 days, or freeze for up to 3 months. If frozen, thaw a container of the hummus in the refrigerator overnight before serving.

✳ **Cooking tip:** A food processor is best for this recipe, so you can drizzle the olive oil in slowly while the motor is running. If you're using a blender, add 1 tablespoon of oil at a time and pulse 5 to 10 times to incorporate.

***Per Serving:*** *Calories: 202; Total Fat: 17g; Saturated Fat: 2g; Protein: 7g; Total Carbohydrates: 8g; Fiber: 4g; Sugar: 1g; Cholesterol: 0mg*

# Roasted Red Potatoes with Herbs

**DAIRY-FREE • GLUTEN-FREE • NUT-FREE • SOY-FREE • VEGAN**
**Makes** 4 servings
**Prep time:** 5 minutes • **Cook time:** 1 hour

These anti-inflammatory roasted red potatoes can be eaten for breakfast, lunch, or dinner. Savory garlic, rosemary, and fresh parsley brighten up this simple side dish and provide numerous antioxidants. The quick and easy, hands-off preparation allows you to work on other meal-prep tasks while the potatoes roast.

---

1½ pounds small red
   potatoes, halved
2 tablespoons olive oil
2 garlic cloves, minced
1 tablespoon chopped
   fresh rosemary
½ teaspoon salt
½ teaspoon freshly
   ground black pepper
2 tablespoons chopped
   fresh parsley

1. Preheat the oven to 400°F. Line a large sheet pan with parchment paper.
2. In a large bowl, combine the potatoes, oil, garlic, rosemary, salt, and pepper and stir gently to coat the potatoes completely. Pour the potatoes and oil mixture onto the sheet pan, scraping any additional oil from the bowl onto the potatoes.
3. Bake for 1 hour, until the potatoes are soft and golden brown with crispy edges, flipping every 20 minutes. Check them at 45 and 50 minutes to make sure they're not getting too brown. Remove them from the oven, set aside to cool, and sprinkle with parsley.
4. Portion the potatoes into 4 medium storage containers.

* **Storage:** Store in the refrigerator for up to 4 days. To serve, microwave the potatoes for 1 to 2 minutes or crisp them back up in the oven (or toaster oven) at 400°F for 5 to 10 minutes.

* **Substitution tip:** Get creative with spices! Feel free to use thyme, chili powder, oregano, or red pepper flakes on the potatoes. You can reduce or increase the amount of garlic according to taste.

*Per Serving: Calories: 182; Total Fat: 7g; Saturated Fat: 1g; Protein: 2g; Total Carbohydrates: 28g; Fiber: 3g; Sugar: 2g; Cholesterol: 0mg*

# Garlic-Lime Black Beans

**DAIRY-FREE • GLUTEN-FREE • NIGHTSHADE-FREE • NUT-FREE • SOY-FREE • VEGAN**

**Makes** 5 servings
**Prep time:** 5 minutes • **Cook time:** 10 minutes

A side of black beans doesn't have to be boring. This recipe is a flavor-packed and versatile staple that goes with so many other dishes in this book. You can whip this up in minutes, using canned beans to save time. You may find yourself wanting to make these beans on every meal-prep day.

1 tablespoon grapeseed
   or coconut oil
1 garlic clove, minced
2 (15.5-ounce) cans
   black beans, drained
   and rinsed
Juice of 1 lime
1 teaspoon ground cumin
½ teaspoon salt

1. In a saucepan, heat the oil over medium heat. Add the garlic and sauté for 1 to 3 minutes, until it starts turning golden brown.
2. Add the black beans, lime juice, cumin, and salt and stir occasionally for 4 to 6 minutes more, mashing some of the beans to create a varied texture. Cool before storing.
3. Portion the beans into 5 storage containers.

✳ **Storage:** Store in the refrigerator for up to 5 days. To serve, microwave for 2 minutes until heated through.

✳ **Substitution tip:** Play with spice levels to taste. Try adding another clove of garlic or adjusting the level of cumin. To give the beans a kick of heat, try adding freshly ground black pepper or hot sauce.

*Per Serving: Calories: 165; Total Fat: 3g; Saturated Fat: 0g; Protein: 9g; Total Carbohydrates: 26g; Fiber: 9g; Sugar: 0g; Cholesterol: 0mg*

# Gluten-Free Tabbouleh Salad

**DAIRY-FREE · GLUTEN-FREE · NIGHTSHADE-FREE · NUT-FREE · SOY-FREE · VEGAN**
**Makes** 6 servings
**Prep time:** 5 minutes · **Cook time:** 10 minutes

This Middle Eastern-inspired dish is a refreshing side that you can serve as a salad, a filling inside a wrap, or even a topping on a burger or salmon cake. The foundation of tabbouleh is parsley, an antioxidant-rich, anti-inflammatory herb. Tabbouleh typically contains bulgur, which is healthy and high in fiber but does contain gluten. Instead, this recipe uses quinoa, which is also high in fiber but is naturally gluten-free.

½ cup quinoa, rinsed
1 cup water
Juice of 1 large lemon
1 garlic clove, minced
⅓ cup olive oil
¾ teaspoon salt
½ teaspoon freshly
   ground black pepper
2 bunches curly parsley,
   leaves and stems,
   finely chopped
½ cup chopped fresh
   mint leaves
2 scallions, thinly sliced
1 medium cucumber,
   seeded and diced

1. In a saucepan, combine the quinoa and water and bring to a boil over high heat. Reduce the heat to medium-low, cover, and simmer for 10 to 12 minutes, until the liquid is absorbed and the quinoa looks fluffy. Remove from the heat and let rest, covered, for 10 minutes more.
2. In a small bowl, combine the lemon juice, garlic, oil, salt, and pepper.
3. In a large bowl, combine the parsley, mint, scallions, and cucumber. Add the warm quinoa and mix to incorporate. Pour the dressing over the entire mixture and gently mix it with a wooden spoon until it is coated.
4. Portion the tabbouleh into 6 medium storage containers or 1 large container.

✱ **Storage:** Store in the refrigerator for up to 5 days.

✱ **Ingredient tip:** Tabbouleh generally contains tomato, so if you're not avoiding nightshades, feel free to add a diced tomato to the mixture.

*Per Serving: Calories: 172; Total Fat: 13g; Saturated Fat: 2g; Protein: 3g; Total Carbohydrates: 12g; Fiber: 2g; Sugar: 1g; Cholesterol: 0mg*

# Cauliflower Herbed Rice

**DAIRY-FREE • GLUTEN-FREE • NIGHTSHADE-FREE • NUT-FREE • SOY-FREE • VEGAN**
**Makes** 4 servings
**Prep time:** 10 minutes • **Cook time:** 10 minutes

Rich and filling but naturally gluten-free and grain-free, this side dish will quickly become a household staple. Cooked with fragrant herbs, this recipe is the perfect way to include more anti-inflammatory vegetables in a way that feels fresh and new. You can "rice" your own cauliflower or, to save time, use refrigerated or frozen riced cauliflower, available at most grocery stores.

1 medium head
  cauliflower, or
  1 (12-ounce) bag frozen
  riced cauliflower
1½ tablespoons
  coconut oil
1 garlic clove, minced
¼ teaspoon salt
¼ teaspoon freshly
  ground black pepper
¼ cup chopped
  fresh basil
¼ cup chopped
  fresh cilantro
¼ cup chopped
  fresh parsley
1 tablespoon finely
  chopped scallions

1. If using whole cauliflower, cut the cauliflower into quarters, remove the stem and core, and "rice" it using the largest holes of a box grater (once grated, the pieces should be the size of grains of rice). If you're using a bag of frozen riced cauliflower, open the bag and set it aside.
2. In a large skillet, heat the coconut oil over medium heat. Add the garlic and cook, stirring often, for 2 to 4 minutes, until it's fragrant and beginning to brown. Add the riced cauliflower and cook, stirring constantly, for 4 to 7 minutes more, until the cauliflower softens and then begins to crisp. Sprinkle with the salt and pepper and stir to incorporate.
3. In a large bowl, combine the basil, cilantro, parsley, and scallions. Add the cauliflower rice and stir gently to incorporate. Cool before storing.
4. Divide the cooled cauliflower rice into 4 medium storage containers.

✳ **Storage:** Store in the refrigerator for up to 4 days, or freeze for up to 2 months. To serve, heat the container in the microwave for 1 to 2 minutes until heated through. If frozen, thaw a container in the refrigerator overnight before reheating.

✳ **Reuse tip:** Cauliflower rice freezes well, so consider making a double batch to use in other recipes, like the Vegetable Fried Cauliflower Rice (page 74).

***Per Serving:*** *Calories: 84; Total Fat: 6g; Saturated Fat: 5g; Protein: 3g; Total Carbohydrates: 8g; Fiber: 3g; Sugar: 3g; Cholesterol: 0mg*

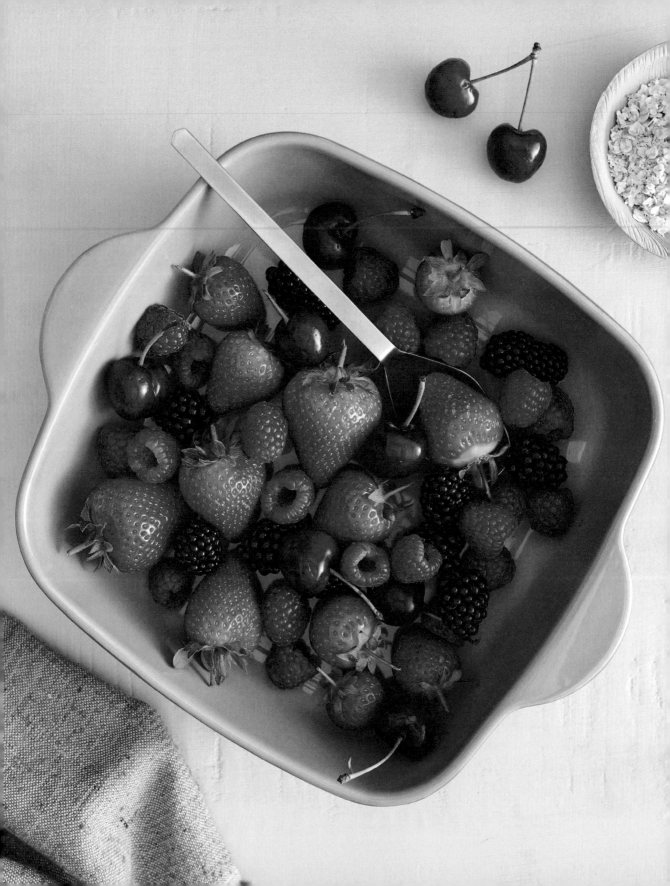

# MEASUREMENT CONVERSIONS

## Volume Equivalents (Liquid)

| US Standard | US Standard (ounces) | Metric (approximate) |
|---|---|---|
| 2 tablespoons | 1 fl. oz. | 30 mL |
| ¼ cup | 2 fl. oz. | 60 mL |
| ½ cup | 4 fl. oz. | 120 mL |
| 1 cup | 8 fl. oz. | 240 mL |
| 1½ cups | 12 fl. oz. | 355 mL |
| 2 cups or 1 pint | 16 fl. oz. | 475 mL |
| 4 cups or 1 quart | 32 fl. oz. | 1 L |
| 1 gallon | 128 fl. oz. | 4 L |

## Oven Temperatures

| Fahrenheit (F) | Celsius (C) (approximate) |
|---|---|
| 250°F | 120°C |
| 300°F | 150°C |
| 325°F | 165°C |
| 350°F | 180°C |
| 375°F | 190°C |
| 400°F | 200°C |
| 425°F | 220°C |
| 450°F | 230°C |

## Volume Equivalents (Dry)

| US Standard | Metric (approximate) |
|---|---|
| ⅛ teaspoon | 0.5 mL |
| ¼ teaspoon | 1 mL |
| ½ teaspoon | 2 mL |
| ¾ teaspoon | 4 mL |
| 1 teaspoon | 5 mL |
| 1 tablespoon | 15 mL |
| ¼ cup | 59 mL |
| ⅓ cup | 79 mL |
| ½ cup | 118 mL |
| ⅔ cup | 156 mL |
| ¾ cup | 177 mL |
| 1 cup | 235 mL |
| 2 cups or 1 pint | 475 mL |
| 3 cups | 700 mL |
| 4 cups or 1 quart | 1 L |

## Weight Equivalents

| US Standard | Metric (approximate) |
|---|---|
| ½ ounce | 15 g |
| 1 ounce | 30 g |
| 2 ounces | 60 g |
| 4 ounces | 115 g |
| 8 ounces | 225 g |
| 12 ounces | 340 g |
| 16 ounces or 1 pound | 455 g |

# REFERENCES

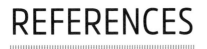

Center for Food Safety and Applied Nutrition. "Final Determination Regarding Partially Hydrogenated Oils." US Food and Drug Administration. FDA. Accessed February 20, 2020. FDA.gov/food/food-additives-petitions/final-determination-regarding-partially-hydrogenated -oils-removing-trans-fat.

Center for Food Safety and Applied Nutrition. "Trans Fat." US Food and Drug Administration. FDA. FDA.gov/food/food-additives-petitions/trans-fat.

Collins, Karen. "Soy and Cancer: Myths and Misconceptions." American Institute for Cancer Research. Accessed March 4, 2020. AICR.org/resources/blog/soy-and-cancer-myths -and-misconceptions.

Craig, M. E., K. W. Kim, S. R. Isaacs, M. A. Penno, E. E. Hamilton-Williams, J. J. Couper, and W. D. Rawlinson. "Early-Life Factors Contributing to Type 1 Diabetes." *Diabetologia* August 27, 2019: 1–2.

Gonzalez de Mejia, E., M. V. Ramirez-Mares, and S. Puangpraphant. "Bioactive Components of Tea: Cancer, Inflammation and Behavior." *Brain, Behavior, and Immunity* 23, no. 6 (2009): 721–31.

Grzanna, R., L. Lindmark, and C. G. Frondoza. "Ginger—An Herbal Medicinal Product with Broad Anti-Inflammatory Actions." *Journal of Medicinal Food* 8, no. 2 (2005).

Heart.org. "How Much Sugar Is Too Much?" Heart.org/en/healthy-living/healthy-eating /eat-smart/sugar/how-much-sugar-is-too-much.

Hlebowicz, J., M. Persson, B. Gullberg, E. Sonestedt, P. Wallström, I. Drake, J. Nilsson, B. Hedblad, and E. Wirfält. "Food Patterns, Inflammation Markers and Incidence of Cardiovascular Disease: The Malmö Diet and Cancer Study." *Journal of Internal Medicine* 270, no. 4 (October 2011): 365–76.

Institute of Medicine of the National Academies. *Dietary Reference Intakes for Water, Potassium, Sodium, Chloride, and Sulfate*. Washington, DC: National Academy of Sciences Press, 2005.

Johnson, R. K., L. J. Appel, M. Brands, B. V. Howard, M. Lefevre, R. H. Lustig, F. Sacks, L. M. Steffen, and J. Wylie-Rosett. "Dietary Sugars Intake and Cardiovascular Health: A Scientific Statement from the American Heart Association." *Circulation* 120, no. 11 (September 15, 2009): 1011–20.

Khan, N., O. Khymenets, M. Urpí-Sardà, S. Tulipani, M. Garcia-Aloy, M. Monagas, X. Mora-Cubillos, R. Llorach, and C. Andres-Lacueva. "Cocoa Polyphenols and Inflammatory Markers of Cardiovascular Disease." *Nutrients* 6, no. 2 (February 2014): 844–80.

Lee-Kwan, S. H., H. M. Blanck, D. M. Harris, and D. Galuska. "Disparities in State-Specific Adult Fruit and Vegetable Consumption—United States, 2015." *MMWR (Morbidity and Mortality Weekly Report)* 66 (2017): 1241–47.

Lefevre, M., and S. Jonnalagadda. "Effect of Whole Grains on Markers of Subclinical Inflammation." *Nutrition Reviews* 70, no. 7 (2012): 387–96.

Liu, Zhao-Min, Suzanne C. Ho, Yu-Ming Chen, Stella Ho, Kenneth To, Brian Tomlinson, and Jean Woo. "Whole Soy, but Not Purified Daidzein, Had a Favorable Effect on Improvement of Cardiovascular Risks: A 6-Month Randomized, Double-Blind, and Placebo-Controlled Trial in Equol-Producing Postmenopausal Women." *Molecular Nutrition & Food Research* 58, no. 4 (2013): 709–17. DOI.org/10.1002/mnfr.201300499.

Noori, N., R. Dukkipati, C. P. Kovesdy, J. J. Sim, U. Feroze, S. B. Murali, R. Bross, D. Benner, J. D. Kopple, and K. Kalantar-Zadeh. "Dietary Omega-3 Fatty Acid, Ratio of Omega-6 to Omega-3 Intake, Inflammation, and Survival in Long-Term Hemodialysis Patients." *American Journal of Kidney Diseases* 58, no. 2 (August 2011): 248–56.

Poti, J. M., M. A. Mendez, S. W. Ng, and B. M. Popkin. "Is the Degree of Food Processing and Convenience Linked with the Nutritional Quality of Foods Purchased by US Households?" *The American Journal of Clinical Nutrition* 101, no. 6 (June 2015): 1251–62.

President's Council on Sports, Fitness & Nutrition. "Physical Activity Guidelines for Americans." HHS.gov. US Department of Health and Human Services. February 1, 2019. HHS.gov/fitness/be-active/physical-activity-guidelines-for-americans/index.html.

Salehi-Abargouei, A., S. Saraf-Bank, N. Bellissimo, and L. Azadbakht. "Effects of Non-Soy Legume Consumption on C-reactive Protein: A Systematic Review and Meta-analysis." *Nutrition* 31, no. 5 (2015): 631–39.

Szabo, G. "Gut-Liver Axis in Alcoholic Liver Disease." *Gastroenterology* 148, no. 1 (January 2015): 30–36.

2015–2020 Dietary Guidelines. Office of Disease Prevention and Health Promotion. Health.gov/our-work/food-nutrition/2015-2020-dietary-guidelines.

Yu, Z., V. S. Malik, N. Keum, et al. "Associations Between Nut Consumption and Inflammatory Biomarkers." *The American Journal of Clinical Nutrition* 104, no. 3 (2016): 722–28.

Zhang H., and R. Tsao. "Dietary Polyphenols, Oxidative Stress and Antioxidant and Anti-Inflammatory Effects." *Current Opinion in Food Science* 8 (April 2016): 33–42.

# RECIPE INDEX

||||||||||||||||||||||||||||||||||||||||||||||||||||||||||||||||||||||||||

# INDEX
||||||||||||||||||||||||||||||||||||||

# ACKNOWLEDGMENTS

This cookbook became possible with the incredible support of many dear friends and family. Trevor, you were with me through those epic grocery shopping trips, and you chopped a lot of onions. A LOT. Your positivity and support mean everything. To my mom, Cheryle, your quality assurance and attention to detail meant your demand to make recipes many times over until they were absolutely perfect. My dad Greg's taste-testing feedback solidified many a recipe in this book. Thank you for supporting this project and for inspiring my passion for cooking as a lifelong activity for me.

I wanted to thank the International Ladies (Cari—and Mark—Jen, Stefanie, Kendra, and Marissa), Julia, Sara, Amy, Brian and Arlo, and Debbie P. I couldn't have done this without you. Thank you to all these friends and the Hultin family for always asking me, "How's the book? When's it coming out?" You pushed me forward, always.

Thank you to Kelly, Kory, Kathleen, Mary, Cynthia, and Debra at Bastyr University for your support of my professional career as well as your ongoing tireless efforts to educate our students, patients, and community about the power of nutrition in healing and wellness.

Thank you to my wonderful agent, Marilyn at O'Shea Literary Agency and to my team at Callisto Media for all their hard work and collaboration on this project.

# ABOUT THE AUTHOR

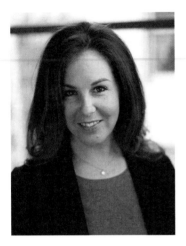

**Ginger Hultin, MS, RDN, CSO**, is a registered dietitian nutritionist and owner of the Seattle-based virtual nutrition practice Champagne Nutrition, where she educates her clients on the balance of including foods they love within a healthy lifestyle. She blogs at Champagne Nutrition and is a national media expert. Her many interviews appear in the *Washington Post*, Food Network, HuffPost, CNN, *Reader's Digest*, and *Wine Spectator,* among many others. She speaks regularly about nutrition and health to large audiences around the world, including recent speaking engagements in Chicago, Illinois; Austin, Texas; Los Angeles, California; Beirut, Lebanon; Amman, Jordan; and Kuwait City, Kuwait.

Ginger completed her undergraduate degree in English literature at the University of Washington and earned a master's degree in nutrition from Bastyr University. A Pacific Northwest native, she resides in the city of Seattle, where she serves as president of the board of her local dietetic association affiliate, the Greater Seattle Dietetic Association. When she's not focused on her nutrition work and volunteer activities, you can find her at her local F45 gym or yoga studio or checking out new neighborhood restaurants.

Ginger believes in the healing power of food and has seen dietary changes alter the course of all her clients' health. Her many years in clinical practice, specializing in nutrigenomics, oncology nutrition, and cardiac health, have led to a passion for educating clients to implement nutrition as part of their care plan. Follow her on Instagram @ChampagneNutrition and on her blog at ChampagneNutrition.com.